The Trust Crisis in Healthcare

The Trust Crisis in Healthcare

CAUSES, CONSEQUENCES, AND CURES

Edited by

David A. Shore

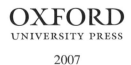

OXFORD

UNIVERSITY PRESS

2007

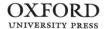

OXFORD
UNIVERSITY PRESS

Oxford University Press, Inc., publishes works that further
Oxford University's objective of excellence
in research, scholarship, and education.

Oxford   New York
Auckland   Cape Town   Dar es Salaam   Hong Kong   Karachi
Kuala Lumpur   Madrid   Melbourne   Mexico City   Nairobi
New Delhi   Shanghai   Taipei   Toronto

With offices in
Argentina   Austria   Brazil   Chile   Czech Republic   France   Greece
Guatemala   Hungary   Italy   Japan   Poland   Portugal   Singapore
South Korea   Switzerland   Thailand   Turkey   Ukraine   Vietnam

Published by Oxford University Press, Inc.
198 Madison Avenue, New York, New York 10016

www.oup.com

Oxford is a registered trademark of Oxford University Press

Library of Congress Cataloging-in-Publication Data

The trust crisis in healthcare : causes, consequences, and cures / edited by David A. Shore.
     p. ; cm
ISBN-13 978-0-19-517636-0
ISBN- 0-19-517636-7
1. Medical care—United States.   2. Trust—United States.   I. Shore, David A.
[DNLM: 1. Delivery of Health Care—United States.   2. Trust—United States.   3. Patient
Satisfaction—United States.   4. Physician-Patient Relations—United States.   W 84 AA1 T873 2006]
RA445.T78 2006
362.10973—dc22

                                                                    2005037264

9   8   7   6   5   4   3   2   1

Printed in the United States of America
on acid-free paper

I dedicate this book to my children, Douglas and Alyssa,
with the hope that the crises of trust in their lives
will be few and far between.

Preface

My deep interest in trust as it relates to healthcare emerged at the conclusion of an address I gave in Washington, D.C., to the *Wall Street Journal* Healthcare Summit. My topic was branding and reputation and the time allocated was 60 minutes. As fate would have it, I finished in 59 minutes, and since a presentation can never be long enough for the speaker, I used my remaining minute to make the observation that the healthcare department, service, institution, or brand that owned trust could own its marketplace. This was followed by a series of rhetorical questions to the healthcare leaders and media in attendance: What would you rather have your organization known for than for being a trusted provider of high-quality services and goods? What would you rather have as your individual legacy than a legacy of trust? If you decided to position yourself around trust, who would your competition be? The level of interest, excitement, and simultaneous discomfort was energizing. The Harvard School of Public Health Trust Initiative was born that day.

What we have learned in the intervening years is that trust is an issue of supply and demand. On the one hand, we suffer from a trust famine, a crisis of trust. On the other hand, the public in general, and health seekers in particular, crave trust in their healthcare providers. A series of trust diagnostics that we have conducted in a wide range of healthcare organizations throughout the United States with a diverse group of stakeholders (i.e., patients, members, physicians, nurses, senior leadership, provider and member relations, nonclinical staff) finds that the question "In your opinion, how important is trust in patient care?" scores as very important or important to all groups. These same stakeholders are equally convinced of the critical importance of trust to the question, "In your opinion, how important is trust to the long-term success of this organization?" Punctuating the data is an episode that occurred just as this manuscript went to press. The evening after conducting a trust diagnostic in a well-known healthcare institution, one stakeholder participant went to dinner with a group of his buddies. During dinner, he discussed the trust diagnostic and proclaimed that he was proud to work for an organization that would choose to invest in trust in such a public way. The next day, one of those buddies at the dinner table applied for a job at that very organization based solely on this testimony. He, too, wanted to work for an organization that placed a premium on trust.

A good number of years have passed since I declared that the healthcare department, service, institution, or brand that could own trust could own its marketplace,

and yet it is perhaps more true today than it was then. Trust is at once good medicine, good business, and great leadership. Most successful organizations attempt
to embrace the FANAFI principle—that is, to find a need and fill it. This book
makes a powerful argument for the need for trust in healthcare and provides some
guidance on how to fill it.

Acknowledgments

I have many thanks to offer. First, my thanks go to Holly Zellweger, my colleague of more than a decade, who has participated in this undertaking every step of the way. It is quite simply a better text thanks to her insight, talent, and dedication. I also thank Eric Kupferberg and Leah Maroni-Wagner for their contributions in finalizing the manuscript. I especially thank John Case, a talented contributor and a very classy human being.

I give special thanks to my editor at Oxford University Press, Carrie Pedersen, who is always accessible and who freed me from many of the usual pressures that come with such an undertaking.

My wife, Charlotte, and my parents, Ruth and Milton, provided the greatest support of all.

Finally, my thanks to all the contributors to this book. I originally had a wish list of "A list" contributors. To my delight, they agreed to participate and gave richly of their time and talent, and we reap the rewards in the pages ahead.

Contents

Contributors

Donald M. Berwick, M.D., M.P.P., is president and chief executive officer, Institute for Healthcare Improvement, a nonprofit organization with projects extending throughout the United States, Canada, Australia, and a number of European countries. A leading national expert on quality in healthcare, he was named by President Clinton to serve on the Advisory Commission on Consumer Protection and Quality in the Healthcare Industry. A clinical professor of pediatrics and healthcare policy at Harvard Medical School, Dr. Berwick has published more than 100 articles in numerous professional scientific journals. In 2005, Dr. Berwick was awarded an honorary KBE (Knight Commander, Order of the British Empire) by Queen Elizabeth II to recognize his "distinguished service to healthcare improvement in Britain's National Health Service."

Robert J. Blendon, M.B.A., M.P.H., Sc.D., M.A., is professor of health policy and political analysis at both the Harvard School of Public Health and the John F. Kennedy School of Government. An expert on public opinion research, he directs the Harvard Opinion Research Program and the Henry J. Kaiser National Program on the Public, Health and Social Policy. Dr. Blendon also codirects the *Washington Post*/Kaiser Family Foundation (KFF) survey project.

Jordan J. Cohen, M.D., is president and chief executive officer, Association of American Medical Colleges, an association that represents all 125 U.S. medical schools, nearly 400 major teaching hospitals, over 90 academic and research societies, and more than 160,000 U.S. medical students and residents. Previously, Dr. Cohen was dean of the medical school and professor of medicine at the State University of New York, Stony Brook, and president of the medical staff of University Hospital. He has also held positions on the medical faculties of the University of Chicago and Harvard, Brown, and Tufts Universities.

Charles M. Cutler, M.D., M.S., is national medical director for quality and clinical integration at Aetna. He is responsible for national quality strategy, clinical function integration, accreditation, patient safety activities, quality measurement and improvement, and serves on Aetna's Racial and Ethnic Disparities Task Force. Prior to joining Aetna, he was the chief medical officer at the American Association of Health Plans, Washington, D.C. He serves on the NCQA's Standards Committee has also served on NCQA's Committee on Performance Measurement. Dr. Cutler has extensive experience in all phases of healthcare operations, health plan benefit design and administration, healthcare policy, and in managing relationships between health plans, employers, regulators, physicians, physician organizations, and other healthcare constituencies.

Michael J. Dowling is president and chief executive officer, North Shore–Long Island Jewish Health System. Prior to becoming CEO, he served as North Shore–LIJ's executive vice president and chief operating officer, and earlier, as senior vice president of hospital services. Dowling also served in the New York State government for 12 years, including two years as a commissioner of social services, and was a longtime chief adviser to Governor Mario Cuomo on health and human services issues.

Howard King, M.D., M.P.H., is a practicing pediatrician and clinical instructor in pediatrics at Harvard Medical School. He is a member of the advisory board for continuing professional education at the Harvard School of Public Health and the Children's Mental Health Task Force for the Massachusetts Chapter of the American Academy of Pediatrics. In 2004–2005, Dr. King directed a funded training program for pediatricians and pediatric nurse practitioners to increase their competence in recognizing psychosocial problems in children and families. He is also developer of a psychosocial Web site for parents and children, Children's Emotional Health-Link. Dr. King was named 2005 Clinician of the Year for the Massachusetts Medical Society (Charles River District). He also received the 2005 Mayor's Medallion Award for Compassionate Health Care.

Greg Koski, Ph.D., M.D., is senior scientist for the Institute of Health Policy and associate professor in the Department of Anesthesiology and Critical Care of the Massachusetts General Hospital at Harvard Medical School. He was the first director of the Office for Human Research Protections, U.S. Department of Health and Human Services, where he gained international visibility and respect for his leadership. He also chaired the Human Subjects Research Subcommittee (HSRS) of the National Science and Technology Council's Committee on Science at the White House and served as executive secretary of the National Human Research Protections Advisory Committee.

Lucian L. Leape, M.D., is adjunct professor of health policy, Harvard School of Public Health. A pioneering researcher in the field of medical errors, he has been one of the nation's leading advocates of the nonpunitive systems approach to the prevention of error and has led several studies of adverse drug events and their underlying systems failures. He was a founding director of the National Patient Safety Foundation and the Massachusetts Coalition for the Prevention of Medical Error. He also led the Institute for Healthcare Improvement's first breakthrough collaborative on the prevention of adverse drug events and was a member of the Institute of Medicine's Quality of Care in America Committee.

Trudy Lieberman is director, Center for Consumer Health Choices, Consumers Union. A journalist for 37 years, she has written about health policy for diverse publications, including

The Nation, Consumer Reports, the *Columbia Journalism Review,* and the *Los Angeles Times.* She has won numerous awards and honors, including two National Magazine Awards, 10 National Press Club Awards, a Fulbright Fellowship to study healthcare in Japan, a John J. McCloy Fellowship to study healthcare in Germany, and a Joan Shorenstein Fellowship at Harvard University to study coverage of medical technology. She is author of five books, including *Slanting the Story: The Forces that Shape the News* (2000).

George D. Lundberg, M.D., is editor-in-chief, Medscape General Medicine; editor-in-chief, Medscape Core; and adjunct professor of health policy, Harvard School of Public Health. From 1982 to 1999, Dr. Lundberg was the American Medical Association's editor-in-chief for Scientific Information and Multimedia and editor of the *Journal of the American Medical Association.* Basically an academic pathologist, he became a medical Internet pioneer in 1995 and in 1999 became editor-in-chief of Medscape, the world's leading Web site for health and medical information; he was founding editor of both Medscape General Medicine and CBS Healthwatch.com. A frequent lecturer and radio and television guest, he is the author of the book *Severed Trust: Why American Medicine Hasn't Been Fixed* (2000).

Marie C. McCormick, M.D., Sc.D., is Sumner and Esther Feldberg Professor of Maternal and Child Health, Harvard School of Public Health, and professor of pediatrics, Harvard Medical School. Her recent awards include election to the Johns Hopkins Society of Scholars as well as election to the Institute of Medicine. She also won the Institute of Medicine's David Rall Medal and the Ambulatory Pediatric Association Research Award. She has served on several advisory and study panels at the Institute of Medicine and was chair of the Institute's Committee on Immunization Safety.

Pippa Norris, Ph.D., is McGuire Lecturer in Comparative Politics, John F. Kennedy School of Government, Harvard University. An expert in elections, public opinion, and political communications, she has published almost three-dozen books and numerous journal articles. Her work has been translated into more than a dozen languages. The most recent books are *Sacred and Secular* (with Ron Inglehart, 2004), *Electoral Engineering* (2004), and *Radical Right* (2005).

Susan P. Pauker, M.D., F.A.C.M.G., is associate professor and a member of the Division of Medical Ethics, Harvard Medical School; chief, Department of Medical Genetics, Harvard Vanguard Medical Associates; and codirector, Massachusetts General Hospital Genetics Clinic. Genetics editor for *Harvard Health Letter*, and *Harvard Women's Health Watch*, Dr. Pauker also serves as clinical geneticist on the board of directors of the American College of Medical Genetics, of which she is a founding fellow.

Cokie Roberts is the chief congressional analyst and a political commentator for *ABC News* and a senior news analyst for National Public Radio. Author of the national bestsellers *Founding Mothers: The Women Who Raised Our*

Nation and *We Are Our Mothers' Daughters,* she is the recipient of the Edward R. Murrow Award and many other broadcasting awards.

Steven V. Roberts is Shapiro Professor of Media and Public Affairs, George Washington University. A *New York Times* correspondent for 25 years, he is a well-known commentator on radio and television. In May 2005 he published a family and childhood memoir, *My Fathers' Houses.* Cokie and Steven Roberts have been married to one another for almost 40 years and are joint authors of a weekly column syndicated by United Media in major newspapers around the country. In February 2000, they published the bestselling book *From This Day Forward,* an account of their marriage and other marriages in U.S. history.

Marc J. Roberts, Ph.D., is symposium cochair and professor of political economy and health policy, Harvard School of Public Health. Author or coauthor of 5 books and 50 articles on healthcare policy and management, environmental policy, and public health ethics, he is widely known as a trainer and consultant in both the United States and abroad. In recent years, he has worked with the governments of China, Hungary, Poland, Bosnia, and Turkey on health sector reform and has taken a leading role in educational programs supported by the World Bank. For 12 years, he served as faculty chairman of the Executive Program for State and Local Public Officials at Harvard.

Dana Gelb Safran, Sc.D., is director of The Health Institute at Tufts–New England Medical Center and Associate Professor at Tufts University School of Medicine. Dr. Safran's empirical research has emphasized the measurement of primary care quality with particular focus on patients' experiences of care and outcomes. By providing detailed and rigorous measurement of the doctor-patient relationship, demonstrating its important influence on outcomes, and highlighting substantial performance variability, Dr. Safran's work has provided an empirical basis for the drive toward inclusion of patients' experiences as essential measures of healthcare quality. Since 1998, Dr. Safran's national studies of Medicare beneficiaries' access to care, quality, and health outcomes have contributed to policy discussions concerning the performance of Medicare HMOs and the debate about prescription drug coverage.

David A. Shore, Ph.D., is associate dean and founding director of the Trust Initiative at Harvard School of Public Health. He teaches two popular Harvard graduate courses, one on strategic marketing and the other on forces of change in the evolving healthcare marketplace. He delivers keynote addresses, presents workshops, and has consulted on six continents. Shore chaired the first three national Conferences on Branding, Positioning, and Competitive Strategies in the Healthcare Industries. His work on brand, reputation, and trust is part of his broader work on market dynamics and the strategies that most powerfully affect the creation of a unique and sustainable competitive advantage. In all of his work, Shore strives to build constructive links between theory and practice. He is the author of *The Trust Prescription for Healthcare: Building Your Reputation with Consumers* (2005).

Richard Toran, M.D., is chief of neurology and medical director, Newton-Wellesley Hospital's Physician-Hospital Organization. Former president of the medical staff at Newton-Wellesley Hospital, he is also an assistant professor of neurology at Tufts University.

Walter C. Willett, M.D., M.P.H., D.P.H., is Fredrick Stare Professor of Epidemiology and Nutrition and chair, Department of Nutrition, Harvard School of Public Health. He has been coinvestigator of the Nurses' Health Study I, principal investigator of Nurses Health Study II, and the Health Professional's Follow-up Study, three large-scale studies designed to investigate the incidence of cancer and other major illnesses. The author of more than 700 articles and a well-known textbook on nutritional epidemiology, he is also author of the best-selling book *Eat, Drink and Be Healthy: The Harvard Medical School Guide to Healthy Eating* (2005).

Christine G. Williams, M.Ed., is director, Office of Communications and Knowledge Transfer, Agency for Healthcare Research and Quality, U.S. Department of Health and Human Services. She is responsible for translating and disseminating the work for the agency to healthcare providers, purchasers, plans, policymakers, consumers, and patients. From 1982 to 1994, Ms. Williams served as senior health policy staff to former Senate Majority Leader George J. Mitchell (D-Maine).

Introduction: Reflections on Trust

COKIE ROBERTS and STEVEN V. ROBERTS

Why, you may ask, would a pair of working journalists write an introduction to a book about the trust crisis in healthcare? Here's one reason: We've been there. After all, most of us in the media rank dismally low on the scale of public trust these days. A recent *USA Today/CNN* poll reports that only 36 percent of Americans express confidence in the media, down from 54 percent 15 years ago. We are right down there with politicians and used-car dealers. Executives of managed-care companies might find our experience useful, since they, too, hover near the bottom of any trust rankings. Even physicians have slipped a bit from their traditionally lofty perch. The healthcare system really has lost much of the trust it once enjoyed, and we know what it's like to be part of an institution that the public regards with a skeptical eye.

But a more serious answer would have two parts. One has to do with the nature of our work. As journalists, we have spent most of our professional careers writing about the people and institutions that govern our society. Trust is a public official's stock in trade, just as it is for any healthcare provider. Only when they command the public's trust can politicians do their jobs effectively. Without it, the work of governing collapses. The bonds between leaders and followers become frayed, the channels of communication filled with static. So our careers in political journalism provide some insight into what the key elements of trust really are—elements that are as important in healthcare as they are in politics.

Then, too, we are members of that vast population that the healthcare system is designed to serve. Other contributors to this volume are healthcare leaders, academic experts, and physicians. We are healthcare consumers, volunteer caregivers, and patients. We have a few thoughts on encountering the various parts of the healthcare system firsthand—and on what causes people to feel both trust and distrust toward healthcare providers.

The Elements of Trust

For all professionals, from politicians and accountants to pastors and healthcare providers, the bond of trust rests on three key foundations: service, candor, and accountability. Take away any one of these elements and trust is compromised. Take away more than one and the bond is ruptured. We have seen such ruptures time and time again in recent years: the corporate misdeeds involving Enron, Tyco, and countless others; the sex abuse scandals in the Catholic Church; the machinations of Wall Street stock analysts; the fabrications and flawed judgments of media figures. Sometimes these scandals cross between professions: The editor of the *Harvard Business Review* was forced out after starting a romantic relationship with a key source—the head of General Electric. The auditing firm Arthur Andersen crumbled after helping Enron cook its books. In both cases, much of the public decided that the institutions in question could no longer be trusted. And now, those who run these stained and strained workplaces face the enormous task of rebuilding that trust.

When institutions *are* trusted, it is because they deliver on those three promises of service, candor, and accountability. Take service first. Service does not merely mean doing something for somebody else. It means delivering *value.* What kind of value do we as professionals offer to those we serve? How is this value perceived by our clients? The perception of value underlies many of the ups and downs in the public's attitude toward government. The high point of trust in the federal government came in the mid-1960s. That was the era of the civil rights movement, the Great Society programs, and the enactment of Medicare. People at the time believed that the government was delivering value—that they were getting their money's worth from their taxes, that their representatives were serving the public interest and not just their own. Within just a few years, however, the Vietnam War and Watergate undermined the public's belief that the government was delivering value. As a result, Ronald Reagan was able to run for president on an antigovernment platform. The federal bureaucracy, in his campaign language, became the "puzzle palace on the Potomac." His popular mantra of attacking "waste, fraud, and abuse" reflected the fact that many people no longer believed that government could provide *them* with valuable services. In fact, they thought government would raise *their* taxes to provide help for others who didn't deserve it. In Reagan's world, the "welfare queen" buying beer with food stamps became the symbol of all that was wrong with Washington.

Trust in the government has waxed and waned since then, as some of the contributions to this book discuss. Ironically, it rose during the Reagan years. The reason is instructive: Even though Reagan ran against the government, he seemed to be delivering on his promises. It fell during the Clinton years, and then rose again after September 11, 2001—partly because voters had confidence in the government's response to terrorism, from the president in the White House to the captain in their local firehouse. But the public also needed government services in a new and personal way—to keep them safe.

The relationship between personal service and public trust is revealed by an interesting fact. People always feel much better about their local representative than about Congress as a whole. In the election of 2002, some 98 percent of the congressional incumbents who sought re-election were successful, a number that is historically quite typical. (Ronald Reagan liked to joke that Congress enjoyed a higher re-election ratio than the Supreme Soviet of the U.S.S.R.—and the Soviets had only one party.) This high rate reflects a critical lesson of governing. As late House Speaker Tip O'Neill would say, all politics is local, and what matters to constituents is often the direct personal service a representative can provide.

For this reason, representatives have vastly increased the staff in their district offices and focused their efforts on direct service. And while that service has a political purpose and payoff, the benefits are totally nonpartisan. It doesn't matter whether you are a Democrat or a Republican. If a lawmaker can help dislodge your mother-in-law's social security check or promote your business deal with some obscure government agency, he or she is delivering value. And the reward is trust. Years ago, Steve saw this change occur in Chester, Pennsylvania, where an aggressive young newcomer named Bob Edgar replaced an aging representative whose only district office was hidden away in a government building and closed most of the time. Edgar opened two storefront offices near mass transit lines and assigned half his staff to casework issues. "There's no overt connection to politics," one of those staffers admitted, "but we recognize there is one."

The same rules and experiences apply to healthcare. Demands are growing for a "patients' bill of rights" because too many clients in health maintenance organizations feel that personal service and consideration are lacking, that too many decisions are made by remote and unaccountable bureaucrats, not people they can meet and talk to, face to face. Ask folks about the rising cost of prescription drugs, and one of the first things they mention is the blizzard of ads on television hawking purple pills for every malady from allergies and indigestion to hair loss and weight gain. And they wonder, Is all that money poured into advertising in my interest? Does it serve me? Or cost me?

The second element of trust is candor. People in Washington always seem to forget—and are doomed to relearn—the aphorism that the cover-up is worse than the crime. Think of the phrases that stick in our memories from the public misdeeds of the last few decades from "I am not a crook" (Nixon) and "I did not have sex with that woman" (Clinton) to Lyndon Johnson's repeated promises that there was "light at the end of the tunnel" in Vietnam. Think of how reluctant the Catholic Church was to acknowledge the transgressions of its priests, or how long it took before brokerage firms admitted that their stock analysts were giving biased information to investors. In all these situations, the public felt, correctly, that it was not getting the straight story and that the people or institutions in question were therefore unworthy of trust. By the same token, consider the admiration with which citizens view politicians such as Senator John McCain or the late Senator Paul Wellstone. Voters who did not agree with all of their policies still admired and supported them because of the quality of their character. Interestingly, both used buses as symbols of their candor and modesty. McCain even dubbed his the "Straight Talk Express" and used it as a rolling stage set for endless press conferences that conveyed this message: I'll answer anything, so you know you can trust me.

Candor allays suspicion. It allows you to release difficult information on your own terms before the media drags it out of you. We've worked in many newsrooms, and we can say with certainty that nothing sets a journalist's antennae quivering quite so keenly as the whiff of a cover-up. Perhaps the worst question any professional can get in any crisis situation is this: What are you trying to hide? Most important, candor represents an investment in building trust, and in fact, a crisis can often be an opportunity to restore and even enhance the public's trust in any institution. Straight talk says to your clients or to your public, "We will tell you everything, even our mistakes. If we screw up, you'll know about it." This is a powerful statement because trust breeds trust. If people know that they can count on you to admit your faults or blunders, if they know you will be candid with them, they will reward your candor with their trust.

The third element of trust is accountability. This is often a sticking point for many professionals. It is the most natural thing in the world to fear accountability. Nobody wants to be exposed in public for his or her misdeeds; nobody wants to pay the price for wrongdoing. But we believe that professionals should welcome mechanisms that hold them accountable. Again, this is an investment that breeds trust.

Take the annual reports by *U.S. News* rating the nation's best hospitals. Many healthcare providers don't like the magazine's ranking system or its methodology— but notice how many institutions in this increasingly competitive marketplace are using those rankings in their advertisements to lure new patients. Hospitals welcome accountability when the news is good and resent it when the news is bad. That's only human nature, but you can't have one without the other. In the end, accountability is a good thing for everybody. It rewards the top performers, prods the underachievers to improve, and convinces the consuming public that the hospitals have nothing to hide.

Consider the situation of the news media. Our relative lack of accountability has long been a sore spot with our readers. They ask us, "Who elected you? What gives you the right to criticize and point fingers?" In recent years, many newspapers have tried to address these concerns. They have established ombudsmen to represent readers' views and reflect their complaints. Some have columnists or reporters who cover the media, including their own employer, often critically. Television news shows criticize newspapers, and newspapers criticize television. Universities produce volumes of media criticism. Granted, this kind of accountability is not the same as having a professional review board or licensing procedure, which in the case of the media would be unconstitutional. But the media have learned that in the absence of outside regulators or certification exams, they need to police themselves, to hold themselves to account. That process can be painful at times, but it's clear that accountability breeds trust rather than undermines it. And healthcare professionals, like journalists, should take the same lesson to heart. If you cannot live with accountability, you do not belong in the business.

In spring 2003, the *New York Times* was hit with a scandal that its own publisher described as a "low point" in the paper's history. A young reporter, Jayson Blair, was caught fabricating dozens of stories and was promptly fired. A few weeks later, the paper published four full pages detailing Blair's misdeeds, a remarkable effort to correct the historical record, but the story had a more significant purpose. It sent a message to *Times* readers: You can trust us to police ourselves, to hold ourselves to high ethical standards. It was a good effort and a good message, but it didn't go far enough. The story tried to pin virtually all of the blame on Blair alone, without detailing the role of *Times* executives who hired

Blair, promoted him despite warnings from their own editors, and created a newsroom culture that permitted and perhaps even encouraged Blair's career as a con man. The story's notable omissions mitigated the impact of its message of trust and left some readers and critics asking that devilish old question, What are they still trying to hide?

The Public's Perspective

As the example of congressional representatives suggests, one factor that affects trust is personal experience with an institution. All of us have some experience with healthcare. We are *consumers*—members of an insurance plan, people who read and think about our health, people who make decisions about our lifestyle and our healthcare. We are *caregivers,* people who take responsibility for caring for children, elderly parents or some other family member, or a friend. And we are *patients,* people who go to the doctor, enter the hospital, or otherwise submit to the ministrations of healthcare professionals.

Like most of the public, we have personal experience with all three roles. And the experiences didn't always build trust. It was women of Cokie's generation who took thalidomide or DES on their doctor's orders, only to find that the drugs could cause birth defects and other problems. They used contraceptive devices such as the Dalkon Shield, which turned out to have unfortunate—sometimes deadly—side effects and then had to fight the manufacturers in court to get compensation for their injuries. More recently, these women have followed hormone replacement therapy regimens, only to be told that these treatments may do more harm than good. Similarly, large numbers of younger women are now taking fertility drugs. No one knows what the long-term effects of these drugs are likely to be on the health of the women and/or their children.

These missteps are in stark contrast to the times when healthcare providers get it right. Diagnostic tests like Pap smears, mammograms, and colonoscopies help detect problems at treatable stages, saving lives and money and strengthening trust in a system that truly cares about its patients. And often, it's the personal touch of one devoted caregiver that makes all the difference. One Easter a few years ago, Steve badly sprained a knee on the tennis court. Our family physician left his own celebration and met us at the hospital emergency room, examined the knee, relieved Steve's pain, and more important, relieved his anxiety. It is a moment we'll never forget, a moment that reinforced the enduring bond of trust between that doctor and our entire family.

Or take the births of our two children. When Cokie went into labor in the middle of the night with the first one, our ob-gyn told us to go to the hospital and then called ahead, warning the staff to expect us. When he found out that an emergency multiple birth was occupying the entire staff, he raced to the hospital, met us when we arrived, and immediately calmed us down. Two years later, when the second child signaled her imminent arrival (we had changed states and doctors by then), our physician refused to believe Cokie when she said that the baby was coming fast. He arrived, as he likes to put it, only in time for the feet, while Steve and the nurse virtually caught our daughter before she hit the floor. Which doctor do we remember fondly? Which one left us with a sense of trust? And which one with a sense of disappointment, even betrayal?

The role of caregiver presents a different sort of trust-related problem. If the patient is elderly, he or she may not want to hear much information from the physician; many people of advanced age simply want the doctor to tell them what to do. But caregivers need information, and they often find that doctors are unwilling to provide it. In one memorable situation, Cokie was caring for the terminally ill husband of a close friend. The friend was away, and the husband's heart stopped. The response of the physician in charge was "We have to restart the heart." Cokie was the only person representing the family, and she wanted to know what else would be involved in the procedure, what the risks were, and what it would mean for the man's life if he revived. The amount of information she could learn at this critical moment was unsatisfactory, and she wound up making the decision to let the doctor proceed only because she was unwilling to take responsibility for not letting them go ahead. In all such situations, it can be very difficult to get the information you need to make appropriate decisions.

Even so, health providers now have to understand that they are dealing with a much more educated group of caregivers who have much more access to information (although not all of it is accurate). Steve had a student whose little brother suffered from a series of disabilities, and no doctor could diagnose or explain the cause. Finally, the child's mother checked his symptoms through various medical texts and journals and arrived at her own conclusion—a certain vitamin deficiency. The doctors reluctantly agreed that she had a point and treated the child for that condition; he has improved dramatically. A young mother we know recently switched pediatricians when her baby wasn't eating properly and her doctor dismissed her concerns out of hand. The lesson: Trust no longer comes automatically with an MD degree. Like other professionals, healthcare providers now have to earn their patient's trust. Every day.

Cokie has been diagnosed with breast cancer and so has recently had intense experience with the role of patient. She has been lucky enough to be cared for at the National Institutes of Health (NIH), where the level of care has been excellent. The physicians at NIH operate with the kind of candor that we mentioned earlier. They also feel no defensiveness when Cokie, as the patient, seeks out other sources of information, whether they are other doctors or the Internet. In fact the NIH staff encourages her research. In that sense they hold themselves accountable: They want their opinions and diagnoses to be checked and supplemented by additional data and other opinions. In all of her time at NIH, Cokie met only one physician who engendered distrust. A callow and intense young man, he continually looked at Steve, rather than at Cokie, while he was trying to convince us to accept a certain treatment regimen. It was an appalling display of insensitivity, and needless to say we turned him down flat. How easy it would have been for that physician to build trust, rather than undermine it, just by directing his attention to the female patient instead of the male relative!

Trust is a matter of big things and little things. It is about the way people set up organizations and institutions to reinforce the three pillars of confidence: service, candor, and accountability. It is also about the way people relate in intimate, one-to-one settings: whether they tell you the full truth, treat you as a human being, and act with respect. Trust in healthcare may be in crisis, and the chapters in this volume analyze and explain causes and consequences of this crisis. But it is a crisis that all of us can help resolve, as long as we understand that trust is earned not given, that it is hard to gain and easy to lose, but that nothing else is more important. We think this book is a great first step in that direction.

I

Trust and Mistrust: The Big Picture

1

The (Sorry) State of Trust in the American Healthcare Enterprise

DAVID A. SHORE

Trust in the professionals and institutions that provide healthcare in America has been eroding over time; indeed, it is now close to an all-time low. The decline in trust seriously compromises medical outcomes, which is a nice way of saying that it endangers patients' lives and well-being. It presents huge challenges to everybody working in the field—clinicians, hospital and managed care administrators and staff, and the manufacturers and marketers of pharmaceuticals and medical devices. It erects a barrier to wise policy-making, both in healthcare and in the public health arena.

This chapter examines the facts that support these contentions. It traces the trends and developments that have led to an erosion of trust, asking where they came from and how they can be reversed. Along with this assessment of the trust landscape, it suggests some methods of eradicating "trust busters," and some methods of encouraging trust builders.[1]

Because "trust" is a word that lends itself to many interpretations, let me first say what I mean by it and explain in a preliminary way why it matters so very much. "Trust is an important lubricant of the social system," wrote Nobel Prize–winning economist Kenneth Arrow in his book *The Limits of Organization.* "It is extremely efficient; it saves a lot of trouble to have a fair degree of reliance on other people's word."[2] In other words, trust facilitates everyday business and social interaction. You do not have to check up on everything people tell you; you assume they will do what they promise to do. What Arrow calls the "invisible institutions: the principles of ethics and morality" constrain individual behavior and encourage trust.[3] (Of course, it helps to have these invisible institutions supplemented by highly visible ones: laws and regulations, police, and courts.)

In healthcare, trust is not merely a lubricant or facilitator, it is an essential part of a well-functioning system. Consider, for example, two everyday experiences with parts of the healthcare system, repeated millions of times a day all over America:

- A patient visits a physician and describes an ailment. The doctor listens to his complaint, examines him, and perhaps runs some tests. Then she offers to write a prescription. The patient goes to the pharmacy, pays a significant amount of money (or expects his insurance company to do so), and ingests the prescribed compound. He is unlikely to know much about what he is ingesting; it is often a chemical substance that would be toxic if taken in large quantities.
- Another patient is admitted to a hospital for surgery. In this case, the experience is more extreme. The patient is stripped naked and knocked unconscious by powerful anesthesia. She is cut open by a surgeon wielding a scalpel, and parts of her body are repaired or removed. Typically, no one other than hospital staff—the surgeon's colleagues and assistants—sees what the doctor does.

Trust, in short, is the bedrock—the very foundation—of healthcare. No thinking person would take any of the actions mentioned unless they had a fundamental level of trust in the professionals with whom they were dealing.

As the examples suggest, trust entails two distinct but equally important elements. If I am to trust you, I must believe that you are competent to do what needs to be done—that you have the necessary skills and resources to do what you say you will do, and that your actions are likely to help me rather than to hurt me. That is why most of us visit a medical doctor rather than a witch doctor when we are sick. I also must believe that you have my best interests at heart and that your judgments and actions are not compromised by a financial (or any other) motive that would put me at risk.[4] To take a particular example, this dimension of trust means that patients can expect their clinicians not to order either too many or too few tests, regardless of financial incentives to err in one direction or the other. Arrow calls this dimension *conscience* and describes it as "essential in the running of society that we have what might be called 'conscience,' a feeling of responsibility for the effect of one's actions on others."[5]

The Erosion of Trust

Americans do have some level of trust in the healthcare system; without it, the system would simply cease to function. But what happens when trust begins to erode? Patients grow nervous and uncertain. They do not know which doctor to see or whether to believe what they are told. They worry about whether they are covered for a given procedure or visit. This compromises the system's effectiveness. Patients, after all, play critical roles in their care. If the care is to be effective, they must take their medication as prescribed, modify their diet, quit smoking, do their physical therapy, and submit to surgery when necessary. Patients who mistrust their doctors are ineffective partners. They don't do what they are supposed to do, and they don't tell their caregivers the truth about what they actually do.

Clinicians are frustrated. Their patients fail to follow instructions. Some sue them for malpractice. At the same time, the managed care companies that provide more and more of clinicians' income put ever increasing restraints on what they can do. Nurses and other caregivers may mistrust the motives and actions of the physicians who are responsible for their patients. Physicians may mistrust the hospitals and other provider organizations to which they refer patients. Stress levels rise all around, and trust suffers.

Healthcare organizations of all sorts find their business models in jeopardy. Pharmaceutical manufacturers, for example, offer patients life-improving and life-saving drugs. Yet they have come under severe attack for what are perceived as their aggressive marketing and pricing policies, and they find themselves subject to strict government regulation. Hospitals receive substantial amounts of money from insurance companies and the government. Yet many find it impossible to operate at a comfortable margin within this system, and most are continually looking for ways to cut costs or minimize services to low-reimbursement patients. Managed care and insurance companies typically pass along their cost increases to their customers, namely employers and employees. But large employers are increasingly concerned about the higher premiums they are being asked to pay, forcing the managed care companies to absorb the increased costs.

The list could go on to include the politics of health policy. What happens, for example, when citizens are "sure" that the cause of high medical costs is insurance company profits? In the public health arena, what happens when no one trusts the government to set rational policies for environmental protection? In all such cases, it becomes harder to mobilize a constituency for effective reform. The erosion of trust is a major problem.

Examining the Data

As my colleague Robert J. Blendon observes in chapter 2, trust in the healthcare system has been on the decline for a while. This broad trend has created a situation where no one has much confidence in the present or, indeed, in the future of the system. Though most Americans trust their own doctors, only 75 percent consider physicians to be the most trustworthy source of healthcare information, and about 50 percent of consumers look to sources other than a doctor for help with healthcare decisions.[6] Only 40 percent of consumers trust hospitals as a source of healthcare information, and still fewer trust healthcare data-collection agencies, employers, government agencies, or insurance companies.[7] Looking to the future, 75 percent of the public believes that hospitals and insurers are not prepared to meet the demands of tomorrow's consumers.[8]

Drill Down into the Data and the Picture Is Still More Troubling

One set of disquieting numbers can be found in the public's opinion of managed care. During the 1990s, the percentage of Americans enrolled in some kind of managed care nearly doubled. While these numbers have declined since 2002, a significant portion of Americans remain covered by this form of insurance.[9] A profound consequence of managed care is an enduring distrust among patients and customers. Surveys conducted at the peak of managed care market penetration

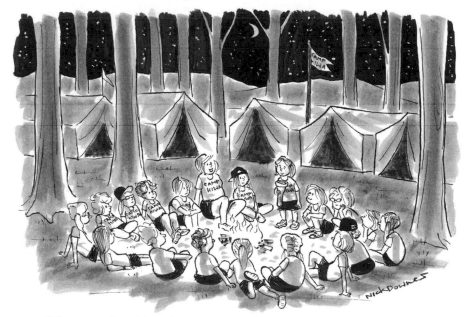

"Very scary, Jennifer—does anyone else have an H.M.O. horror story?"

Figure 1.1. Distrust in HMOs

Source: Nick Downes, "Very scary, Jennifer—does anyone else have an H.M.O. horror story?" [Cartoon.] *The New Yorker*, July 19, 1999. Available: http://www.cartoonbank.com (accessed April 19, 2006).

revealed that nearly half of enrollees viewed managed care as a bad thing. Slightly more than half believed that it threatened the quality of care. Only a third predicted that managed care would make their health plans more responsive to them as customers.[10] Healthcare expert and author Paul H. Keckley summarizes the situation well: "Most providers and consumers do not trust health plans, especially for quality of care decisions. In fact, for most patients the prevailing notion is that plans exist to restrict their choices of providers and limit their options for care to the cheapest rather than the best."[11] The verdict calls to mind a *New Yorker* cartoon (Figure 1.1) in which a group of children at camp are gathered around the campfire, and one has just finished telling a story. "Very scary, Jennifer," says the counselor. "Does anyone else have an HMO horror story?"

A second set of data derives from the fact that people's level of trust in the healthcare system varies dramatically with age, gender, geography, socioeconomic status, and their own health. Low-income patients trust it less than higher-income patients. Those who are in poorer health trust it less than those who are in better health.[12] Such disparities exist even when different cohorts have the same insurance coverage. Nor does the story end there. Racial and ethnic minorities are almost twice as concerned as the general population about errors when they receive healthcare.[13] African-Americans and Latinos are less likely to have visited a doctor in the past year than their Caucasian counterparts, and they are less likely to have a regular healthcare provider. Startlingly, although 51.4 percent of *uninsured* Caucasians say they have a regular healthcare provider, the percentage drops to 18.4 percent for African Americans and 20.3 percent for Latinos. Can people trust a system in which they don't fully participate?[14]

To be sure, the trust picture is not uniformly bleak. Most Americans—the figure hovers around 90 percent—continue to trust their own doctors.[15] (As with representatives in Congress, it is all the others that they don't trust.) And year-to-year changes sometimes show small improvements in public attitudes. For instance, in 2005 more than three-quarters of Americans—79 percent—felt that hospitals were doing a good job; that figure was up from 70 percent in 2004. Forty-one percent felt that managed care companies were doing a good job in 2005; that figure was up from 30 percent the previous year.[16] But it would be unwise to put too much faith in the occasional positive indicator or in modest year-to-year fluctuations. Too many other indicators suggest a serious lack of trust over time. An analysis of where and why trust is eroding is not encouraging to those who hope that the problem will simply go away.

What Contributes to the Decline?

The erosion of trust in healthcare during the past few decades is partly attributable to society-wide trends. The social movements that began in the 1960s generated a deep and abiding mistrust of institutions in general and of science in particular. As other chapters in this book show, trust in everything from the U.S. government to the media has been on the wane. In this respect, healthcare has merely been swept along by the wave of declining trust. The collective of women who wrote *Our Bodies, Ourselves* in the 1970s argued that the male-dominated medical profession could not be trusted to oversee childbirth or breast-cancer treatment without engaging in demeaning and destructive treatment of women's bodies.[17] The book's popularity was as much a cultural phenomenon as a medical one.

But developments within healthcare itself contributed mightily to the decline in trust. Three in particular stand out: the change in the dominant delivery system; the accompanying change in the model of the patient-doctor relationship; and the new self-scrutiny of the medical profession, leading to widespread publicity about patient safety and medical errors.

The New Delivery System

People who came of age in the middle decades of the twentieth century grew accustomed to a remarkably simple healthcare system. When they were sick, they went to a doctor. They paid him (and it was usually a man) in cash, or if they were covered by insurance, the plan automatically reimbursed him. If they needed hospitalization, they were admitted to a hospital, which typically had plenty of available beds. The costs of the system were relatively low. Doctors enjoyed high social status and even higher levels of trust. Hospitals were prestigious local institutions, heavily supported by philanthropy. Medicare and Medicaid, introduced in the 1960s, extended government insurance coverage to the elderly and the poor, thereby ensuring that the vast majority of Americans had access to the system.

In recent years, a variety of factors have conspired to undermine this model. Increasing use of expensive new technologies and pharmaceuticals pushed up the cost of treatment. High demand for services—coupled with generous insurance coverage—allowed providers to raise their fees. As costs rose across the board, health maintenance organizations and other forms of managed care appeared. Suddenly, people found themselves in situations where a variety of gatekeeping devices limited their access to care. They could no longer choose their doctor or hospital. They could no longer get automatic access to specialists. Reimbursements for various treatments were constrained by formularies and fine print.[18] Women who once might have spent a week or two in the hospital after childbirth were now ushered out the next day in a practice appropriately dubbed "drive-through delivery."

Along with managed care came the rise of the for-profit healthcare sector. Hospitals in the past had nearly always operated on a not-for-profit basis; so, too, did Blue Cross Blue Shield, the primary health insurer for many Americans. But many of the new managed care organizations, hospitals, and medical groups were now profit-seeking businesses. Increasingly, patients realized that providers and insurers might have interests that were at odds with their own and that the pressure to please investors could lead for-profit firms to act on those interests.[19] Press reports of high profits, rising stock prices, and generous executive compensation fueled the mistrust. So, too, did the intensified competition among hospitals and other healthcare providers, which led even the old nonprofits to pursue much more businesslike, cost-efficient practices. While this often had positive effects, it made going to the hospital a more complex experience than it had been. Indeed, the effects were not always positive. A study reported in the *Journal of the American Medical Association,* for instance, reported that the risk of dying after surgery jumps 14 percent when a patient's nurse has six beds to cover rather than four. It soars by more than 30 percent if the nurse is responsible for eight beds.[20]

The New Patient-Doctor Relationship

Another characteristic of the mid-twentieth-century system was that the doctor was very much in charge. He dispensed advice, prescriptions, and other treatment, and he did not expect to be questioned or challenged. How could patients do so, anyway? They were not medically trained. If information is power, the doctor had all the information, hence all the power. The story is told of the man who arrived at the pearly gates and saw an imposing figure with a stethoscope draped around his neck. "Is that a doctor?" the man asked. "No," St. Peter replied—"that's God. He likes to play doctor." It was a wry commentary on the common opinion that doctors consider themselves to have god-like powers.

However, a variety of factors undermined this model. The social movements of the 1960s encouraged people to "question authority," as the popular bumper sticker put it, and the doctor's presumed expertise was questioned as much as that of other authority figures. Consumer-oriented organizations and publications began evaluating the efficacy of various treatments and publicizing the information. Managed care also challenged the physician's authority. Suddenly, what the doctor ordered might be subject to review and approval by another physician or even a nurse working for the managed care company. In recent years, of course, patients have realized that they can gather huge amounts of information (and misinformation) about their illnesses or injuries from the Internet, and they often come to the doctor's office with distinct ideas about what kind of treatment they prefer. They are also likely to bring information from a direct-to-consumer (DTC) advertisement from a pharmaceutical company—saying, in effect, "I want this one"—and in the majority of cases physicians give them what they want. Doing so keeps the patient happy and invested in the treatment, and it takes less time than talking them out of what they want and into something that might be more effective. The result of all this is that the fundamental relationship between patient and doctor is changing from *compliance* to what might be called *concordance*. The patient is no longer a passive partner; he or she typically seeks to be an active one.

On balance, this is far from a bad thing. It is the patients, after all, who play the most important part in determining their health. Their attitude toward treatment and their behavior (e.g., taking medication) goes far toward determining the likely efficacy of the physician's recommendations. Indeed, many in healthcare today suggest that their mission is to help people *manage* their *own* health. From a trust perspective, the new model cuts both ways. Physicians are often scornful of patients' desire to play a role and often fall back on the old "do as I say" model—a trust buster, if there ever was one. Often dangerously armed with a little knowledge, patients may decide that doctors don't know what they're talking about and hence cannot be trusted. As with any change, the destination may be desirable, but there are many bumps and potholes along the way.

Medical Errors

The subject of medical errors—always controversial, always scary—is discussed at greater length elsewhere, notably in chapter 5 by Dr. Lucian L. Leape, a pioneering researcher in the field. But no survey of the trust landscape can ignore it, because medical errors (and publicity about them) are a major factor in the erosion of trust.

We do not know the exact magnitude of the problem. A study from the Institute of Medicine—extensively quoted and challenged—says that medical errors are responsible for 44,000 to 98,000 deaths per year.[21] Dr. Leape uses the figure 180,000, and estimates that two-thirds of total deaths are preventable. Others claim that there are at least 225,000 deaths per year caused by medical errors and adverse effects, which would place iatrogenic events third in causes of death, after heart disease and cancer. Barbara Starfield, in an article in the *Journal of the American Medical Association,* breaks this number down to include the following:

- 12,000 deaths per year from unnecessary surgery
- 7,000 deaths per year from medication errors in hospitals
- 20,000 deaths per year from other errors in hospitals
- 80,000 deaths per year from nosocomial infections (those originating in hospitals)
- 106,000 deaths per year from non-error adverse effects of medication.[22]

Note that these estimates are for deaths only; they do not include errors or adverse effects that lead to discomfort or disability.

For our purposes, the exact number of deaths due to error is not central. It is enough to note that the number is large and has generated a huge amount of coverage in the media and hence in patients' minds. Responsible reports of errors are often overshadowed by the sensational. One rather startling event was the placement in mid-2001 of a two-page ad in six consumer magazines, including *People, Parents,* and *Family Circle.* The ad featured a pie chart titled "Major Causes of Death in the United States." It had a slice for breast cancer, a slice for vehicular accidents, and a slice for AIDS (autoimmune deficiency syndrome). The fourth slice, nearly as large as the other three together, was simply for "Oops!" The chart's caption warned healthcare consumers of the dangers of medical errors. It then provided eight practical tips to help consumers prevent them. Within the healthcare field, the ad sparked controversy about its facts and presentation. Nevertheless, from the perspective of impact on the public, this was a landmark ad, in that a major player in the industry and a company widely regarded as an innovator—UnitedHealth Foundation, a foundation sponsored by UnitedHealth Group—was publicizing the claim that medical errors are both widespread and serious. When a major company in the industry runs an ad such as this, the public can hardly be blamed for thinking that physicians, managed care, and hospitals are more likely to harm them than to help them. A comparison of accidental gun deaths with deaths caused by medical error has appeared on hundreds of Web sites and in chain e-mails.[23] The compiled statistics suggest that the number of iatrogenic deaths per doctor in the United States vastly exceed the number of accidental gun deaths per gun owner. If this compilation is to be believed, doctors are approximately 9,000 times more dangerous than gun owners! This type of public dialogue both reflects and reinforces the downward spiral of trust in healthcare.

The Role of the Media

The erosion in trust is a self-perpetuating cycle: The more consumers come to distrust the healthcare system, the more aware they are of every fact or allegation that seems to confirm the distrust. In effect, they believe that the news reports the norm, and the media and popular culture reinforce this view.

On television, the kindly and trustworthy physician on *Marcus Welby M.D.* has been replaced by the laughable characters on sitcoms such as *Scrubs* and by the valiant medical professionals on shows such as *ER,* where the doctors often battle against an uncooperative bureaucracy and insurance system. Television medical dramas in 2001 featured an average of one scene per episode that discussed a public policy healthcare issue. Here are some examples:

- In an episode of the popular Lifetime show *Strong Medicine,* a critically ill, low-income patient learns that she doesn't have access to the prescription drugs she needs because her inner city neighborhood isn't adequately served by the major pharmacies.
- In the ABC drama *Gideon's Crossing,* a woman learns that her leukemia was misdiagnosed by her overworked and possibly careless HMO doctor.
- In an episode of *ER,* an HMO won't allow a woman with terminal breast cancer to be admitted to the hospital for pain management.

A study by the Kaiser Family Foundation of these and other television treatments of healthcare issues found that the shows generally did not tilt either for or against the status quo in their portrayal, but they did reference most of the leading institutional players in the health policy debates, including hospital administrators, lawyers, government agencies, insurance companies, and HMOs. Of these, three groups tended to be cast as villains: insurance companies, lawyers, and HMOs. Indeed, every single reference to HMOs during the 2000–2001 television season was negative.[24] The impact of such consistent depiction is substantial. Television dramas reach a much wider audience than news shows, and in many ways they are even more powerful. Vicky Rideout, a vice-president of the Kaiser Family Foundation, which oversaw the study, says, "Instead of bill numbers and budget figures, health policy issues are portrayed through the lives of characters the viewer cares about, often in life or death situations."[25]

No clearer example of the power of popular culture could be found than the movie *John Q,* released in 2002 by New Line Cinema. In the film, a young boy named Michael needs a heart transplant. Michael's father—John Q. Archibald, played by Denzel Washington—learns that his insurance company doesn't cover the procedure. The hospital demands a $75,000 cash payment in advance. Archibald does not have the money, and the movie is about the desperate measures he takes to try to get his son the medical attention he needs to survive. It is fiction, to be sure, but it is based on a true story, and John Q. is one of the more sympathetic characters to grace the big screen in recent years.

The subtext is as important as the text. John Q. assumes that his HMO would cover whatever treatment his son needed. (Why else would you have health insurance if not for circumstances like this?) Among those who had heard of the movie, more than 7 in 10 said they believe real life insurers refuse to pay for treatments like this. About 4 in 10 think this happens "a lot," while 3 in 10 believe it happens "sometimes."[26] In response to *John Q,* the American Association of Health Plans announced in the summer of 2002 that it had retained Hollywood's leading talent agency, William Morris, in an effort to "build bridges between health plans and the entertainment community." However well intended the association's effort may have been, can consumers be faulted for regarding such a move cynically?[27]

Another source of distrust has been the public health arena. For years, Americans were told to believe in the food pyramid constructed by the U.S. Department of Agriculture, which ostensibly shows how much of different food groups constitute a healthy diet. Now we learn that the food pyramid may have been highly misleading, not to say downright wrong. (Readers will learn more in chapter 12 by Walter Willett, the Harvard School of Public Health physician whose research has contributed mightily to the rethinking of the pyramid.) But this is only the latest in a series of seeming public health reversals by researchers, academics, and policy makers. Middle-aged women flocked to hormone replacement therapy, for example, only to learn from new research (in 2002) that the risks may outweigh the benefits. A major study of medicine for hypertension found that older drugs, diuretics, may be more effective than newer ones. Yet the newer ones were heavily marketed by their manufacturers and largely replaced the older products.[28]

As Dr. Willett points out, it comes as no surprise to a scientist that one set of findings should be overturned by new information. These conflicts and contradictions "are the way science works . . . Men and women carry out studies and report their results. Evidence accumulates. Like dropping stones onto an old-fashioned scale, the weight of evidence gradually tips the balance in favor of one idea over another."[29] But the popular media put quite a different interpretation on the contradictory studies. According to most media stories, the researchers got it "wrong" the first time and claim they are getting it "right" now. The implication: Why should anyone believe them?

The Docket of Distrust

The result of these changes, medical and cultural, is a toxic atmosphere in which nobody puts much trust in anybody else. The docket of distrust is long—too long.[30]

- Consumers who belong to managed care plans do not trust the plans to make decisions based on medical necessity rather than cost. "Managed care is winning in the healthcare marketplace, but is in danger of losing the battle for public opinion," said Drew E. Altman, president of the Kaiser Family Foundation.[31] The comment was made some time ago, but the point holds true today.
- Consumers do not trust hospitals to look out for their best interests, either. Too often the first question hospitals greet patients with is "What is your insurance?" rather than "How can we help you?" Hospital bills are too high, and incomprehensible, in most consumers' opinion.
- Physicians distrust managed care plans as much as consumers do. In fact, many report that they manipulate reimbursement rules and otherwise game the system to get coverage for procedures they deem necessary. Doctors are rarely shy about making it clear who denied a particular claim. After all, it makes them look like the good guys.

- Many referring physicians don't trust hospitals; they fear that the hospital is trying to "steal" their patients. And all physicians with hospitalized patients worry about the possibility of medical error or other iatrogenic event. Physicians do not greatly trust pharmaceutical companies or medical device manufacturers, either.
- Nurses don't trust many physicians, whom they experience as high handed or worse; physicians are often accused by nurses of abusive treatment or sexual harassment. Nurses also do not trust hospital administrations, believing that, if they really wanted to do something about staffing ratios and workloads, they would.
- Managed care companies, for their part, may not trust their physicians or members to play by the companies' rules. They also have little trust in pharmaceutical companies, whom they accuse of overcharging for products and pandering to customers' hopes and fears through direct-to-consumer advertising. A proprietary study done in 2001 by a major pharmaceutical company revealed that managed care medical directors characterized the industry as "aggressive," "greedy," "self-serving," and "not to be trusted."
- In a supreme irony, the more financially successful healthcare businesses are *less* likely to be trusted by consumers. In 2000, for example, HMOs generally registered healthy profits—and were confronted by the suspicion that profits were achieved by the industry's "dumping" high-cost or low-paying members.[32]

Thus the trust problem of the healthcare system is the moral equivalent of a chronic condition. All the personal experiences and all the cultural reinforcements build on one another and reinforce the impression that a system seemingly composed of profit-obsessed corporations, overstressed doctors, and large impersonal institutions is not as trustworthy as the perhaps mythical family doctor of the Marcus Welby era.

The Search for Solutions

Can anything be done about this erosion of trust in healthcare? The question, of course, is the explicit or implicit subject of most of the chapters in this book. At the most fundamental level, high levels of trust promote better medical outcomes at lower cost. Patients who trust their doctors and other providers become active partners in their care. They do what they are supposed to do and do not do what they aren't supposed to do.[33] Clinicians who trust one another work together smoothly and do not waste time bickering. They also waste less time practicing defensive medicine, such as ordering tests that may be medically unnecessary but could serve to ensure against a possible lawsuit. Trust is *efficient,* as Kenneth Arrow observes. It lowers costs by allowing everybody to focus on the problem, rather than on checking up on each other. It also allows patients to have confidence in people and institutions that they may otherwise be unqualified to judge. A doctor or hospital—even, in theory, a managed care company—that earns my trust thereby earns the right to make decisions on my behalf, without having to walk me through every possible alternative. Thus trust reduces costs in part by accelerating the sales and utilization cycle.

There are two other reasons—one negative, one positive—why healthcare providers and organizations need to build trusting relationships among their clientele. First, trust is simply too important in healthcare to be ignored. If consumers believe that they cannot trust healthcare providers, they will demand that government agencies step in to regulate the business even more closely. Take, for example, the previously mentioned study that reported that patients' risk of dying after surgery increases noticeably when nurses are responsible for more beds. Can consumers be blamed if they feel a little nervous, particularly when they read headlines such as "Nursing Shortage Can Have Deadly Consequences"? In response, the state of California passed a law in 2004 mandating nurse-to-patient ratios in all parts of the hospital: one for every six medical or surgical patients, and one for every two emergency department patients in critical care.[34] Many more such regulations are likely to be legislated, unless healthcare providers can rebuild a level of trust that makes further government action unnecessary.

Second, trust is a critical factor for anyone who wants to build a successful business in the healthcare industry. The trusted physician attracts and keeps his or her patients; indeed, trust is the single biggest predictor of patient loyalty to a physician's practice. The trusted hospital attracts not only the best clinicians but also the most patients and the most donors (or investors). The trusted managed care company or pharmaceutical manufacturer can gain market share at its competitors' expense. Think of names such as Mayo Clinic, Massachusetts General Hospital, Blue Cross Blue Shield, Johnson & Johnson, or GE Medical Systems. It is hardly an exaggeration to say that the organization that owns trust owns its marketplace. Consumers frequently say that they purchase something simply because it carries a brand that they trust. When that "something" is a person's medical care, the frequency is undoubtedly significantly higher.

Rebuilding Trust

Suppose providers and healthcare organizations were to adopt the building of trust as a guiding principle, their North Star. What steps would they take?

Service Quality

It goes without saying that they would need to establish and monitor high levels of quality. But quality in a service industry such as healthcare is a complex matter. It includes obvious and critical measures such as low levels of medical errors (see chapters four and five by Drs. Berwick and Leape, respectively). It also includes dozens—maybe hundreds—of other indicators, many intangible, many difficult to measure and manage. Is the receptionist pleasant? Does the physician's or surgeon's manner encourage trust? Is billing handled professionally and courteously? Is the physical environment clean and well maintained? Sometimes seemingly trivial factors have large and demonstrable impacts on perceptions of quality, hence on trust. If a hospital's parking lot is poorly managed or unsafe, patients are likely to have less confidence in the quality of its other services. If the wastebasket in the washroom is overflowing, patients (and their families) may assume that the rest of the facility isn't very clean, either. All of these quality indicators, moreover, must be the same day after day, month after month, visit after visit, year after year. Any company with a great brand—what I call a *power brand*—obsesses about consistency.[35]

Consistent high quality and trust building is necessary across the board. If members of a managed care company cannot get a courteous customer service representative on the phone, the members are unlikely to trust the company. If consumers believe that a pharmaceutical manufacturer is overcharging or otherwise bilking its customers, no matter how good the company's drugs are, they won't trust it. A commitment to building trust has to permeate an organization. Merely to make this observation is to acknowledge how much work remains to be done in most organizations.

Responsiveness

Trust-seeking organizations must be learning organizations. They must learn from experience what builds trust and what destroys it. Some companies, for instance, have learned that rigid gate keeping is one of the facets of managed care that most aggravates clinicians and consumers; in response, they have loosened their controls considerably. Dr. Dana Safran (see chapter 7) has found that consumer trust in health maintenance organizations varies considerably with the structure of the organization, especially the degree to which the organization is seen to restrict choice and physician independence. The more access consumers have to the doctors they want to see—and the more those doctors can make decisions or referrals without worrying about a gatekeeper—the more likely everybody will trust the HMO.

The real test of responsiveness comes when an adverse event occurs. There is a saying in Washington, D.C.: "You don't get in trouble for the deed, you get in trouble for the cover-up." And a remarkable number of healthcare organizations do try to cover up adverse events, whether it is a highly visible medical error or simply a poor report card. Compare that behavior with the way Johnson & Johnson (J&J) handled the tragedy of Tylenol laced with cyanide. The company recalled millions of dollars of the drug. Chief Executive Officer Jim Burke went on television and told the public exactly how the company was responding. The forthright strategy won J&J the distinction of having the "best crisis management campaign of the twentieth century." They also won back their market share in record time.[36] Amazingly, the Tylenol lesson often goes unlearned.

Brand Identity

"Brand" is a word that many people in the healthcare industry find distasteful. It smacks of commercialism, advertising, marketing—appropriate to other industries, but not to healthcare. (Of course, pharmaceutical and medical-device manufacturers, along with for-profit healthcare providers, do not typically share these concerns.) But whatever the feelings, any healthcare provider or organization does have a brand, and that brand means something to people. "Brand image" is *what* the marketplace perceives. "Brand identity" is the *desired* marketplace perception. The two are not always synonymous. In its early days, for example, Kaiser Permanente Health Plans was known for providing adequate care, a sort of Hyundai of the healthcare market, respectable but hardly top of the line. And the assessment was more or less accurate, in part because Kaiser didn't attract cream-of-the-crop clinicians. (When physicians referred to "Kaiser doctors," it was not a compliment.) Today, Kaiser is by most measures a high-quality provider. But its brand image has scarcely changed; it is often still thought of as a Hyundai.

What does this brief lesson in marketing have to do with trust? Just this: It doesn't do you any good to be high quality if you're not *perceived* to be high quality, that is, if you're not trusted. In that sense, perception is reality. And perception depends not only on facts and logic but, as Aristotle reminds us, on emotions. That means using all the tools and techniques of branding to build a power brand. In healthcare, there aren't yet many power brands (see chapter 15).[37]

A Turning Point?

Healthcare is at a tipping point. My hope is that it will also represent a turning point. Right now, healthcare consumers (like citizens in general) are experiencing what journalists call the "mean world" syndrome. The news seems always bad. Trust is constantly eroding. It is a vicious cycle in which improvements may not be noticed because the bad news makes the headlines and confirms consumers' fears. But often a virtuous cycle follows a vicious one. Positive experiences add up; the bad news begins to seem more like the exception than the rule; the assumption that the system can be trusted after all becomes widely held. This has happened throughout history, and then the whole thing is forgotten because the new state of affairs is taken for granted. For example, most of us don't remember the rampant corruption among metropolitan police forces a century ago. Then, corruption was the norm. Today, it is perceived by most to be the exception. But it was a long hard road to get to where we are today.

In healthcare, the road may not need to be either so long or so hard. The pendulum has swung from blind trust to deep suspicion; the laws of physics suggest that it may already be on its way back toward the middle. Everybody has an interest in building trust: patients, clinicians, organizations, government. Everybody will benefit from increasing levels of trust. The problem is being named and analyzed, and solutions are being offered. Providers and healthcare organizations can pick these up and run with them. Tom Schultz, a healthcare executive with whom I worked closely during his tenure at the Baptist Health System (Alabama), puts it this way: "The healthcare industry has an opportunity to be leaders in building trust in a world that is becoming more cynical" (personal communication, December 18, 2005). I am not sure whether that is best called a mission or a vision—but either way, it is a worthy objective.

Notes

1. For an expanded discussion of these several themes, see David A. Shore, "The Current State of Trust in the American Healthcare Enterprise," (White Paper, 2004), 1–18; and David A. Shore, *The Trust Prescription for Healthcare* (Chicago: Health Administration Press, 2005). Many of these remarks are echoed in Alice K. Jacob's 2004 Presidential Address before the meeting of the American Heart Association, "Rebuilding an Enduring Trust in Medicine: A Global Mandate," *Circulation* 111 (2005): 3494–3498.

2. Kenneth J. Arrow, *The Limits of Organization* (New York: Norton, 1974), 23.

3. Arrow, *Limits of Organization,* 26.

4. For an extended examination of the nature of trust in healthcare and in other social realms, see Lucy Gilson, "Trust and the Development of Health Care as a Social Institution," *Social Science & Medicine* 56 (2003): 1453–1468, esp. 1454–1459.

5 Arrow, *Limits of Organization,* 27.

6. VHA Inc. and Deloitte & Touch LLP, "Healthcare 2001: A Strategic Assessment of the Healthcare Environment in the United States," in *2002 AHA Environmental Assessment* (Chicago: American Hospital Association, 2002), reprinted in *Hospitals & Health Networks* 76 (Sep 2002).

7. VHA Inc. and Deloitte & Touch LLP, "Healthcare 2001."

8. Pricewaterhouse Coopers, "Healthcare Practice," in *2002 AHA Environmental Assessment* (Chicago: American Hospital Association, 2002).

9. *Trends and Indicators in the Changing Health Care Marketplace* (Menlo Park, Calif.: Kaiser Family Foundation, 2002), 17; D. A. Draper et al., "The Changing Face of Managed Care," *Health Affairs* 21 (Jan/Feb 2002): 11–23; M. Susan Marquis et al., "The Managed Care Backlash: Did Consumers Vote with their Feet?" *Inquiry—Excellus Health Plan* 41 (Winter 2004/2005): 376–390; and, David Mechanic, "The Rise and Fall of Managed Care," *Journal of Health & Social Behavior* 45 (Dec 2004): 76–86. Despite the gradual decline in national numbers, managed care systems remain prominent in some states (*e.g.*, California) and in many Medicaid programs. See, "HMO Penetration 2000 and 2003 in the 10 Most Populous States," *Healthcare Financial Management* 59 (Nov 2005): 11; and, Debra Draper, Robert E. Hurley, and Ashley C. Short, "Medicaid Managed Care: The Last Bastian of the HMO?" *Health Affairs* 23 (Mar/Apr 2004): 155–168. Some authors have predicted a return of managed care arrangements, in part to combat the continued rise in healthcare costs. See, Glen P. Mays, Gary Claxton, and Justin White, "Managed Care Rebound? Recent Changes in Health Plan's Cost Containment," *Health Affairs* 23 (Jul–Dec 2004): 427–437.

10. "More Evidence That Backlash Against Managed Care Has Bottomed Out; Image May Be Improving Slightly," *Harris Interactive Healthcare News* 1:23 (July 30, 2001), 1–3. Available: http://www.harrisinteractive.com/news/newsletters/healthnews/HI_HealthCareNews2001V011_iss23.pdf (Accessed March 31, 2006). American HMO enrollees have been particularly troubled by the seeming loss of autonomy with regard to selecting providers, hospitals, and treatments. See, Daniel Simonet, "Patient Satisfaction Under Managed Care," *International Journal of Health Care Quality Assurance* 18 (2005): 424–440; B. M. Jennings et al. "What Really Matters to Healthcare Consumers," *Journal of Nursing Administration* 35 (Apr 2005): 173–180; D.E. Grembowski et al., "Managed Care and Patient-Rated Quality of Care from Primary Physicians," *Medical Care Research and Review* 62 (Feb 2005): 31–55; and, Jennifer S. Haas et al., "Is the Prevalence of Gatekeeping in a Community Associated with Individual Trust in Medical Care?" *Medical Care* 41 (2003): 660–668.

11. Paul H. Keckley, "Evidence-Based Medicine: The Strategic Framework for Reinventing Health Plans," n.d. Available: http://bcbshealthissues.com/proactive/newsroom/releast.vtml?id-33923 (accessed June 4, 2003).

12. See Pippa Norris, "Skeptical Patients: Performance, Social Capital, and Culture," in this volume for a discussion of other differences. V. B. Sheppard, R. E. Zambrana, and A. S. O'Malley provide a discussion of the dimensions of trust among low-income women and their healthcare providers in "Providing Health Care to Low-Income Women: A Matter of Trust," *Family Practice* 21 (2004): 484–491.

13. The Kaiser Family Foundation and the Agency for Healthcare Research and Quality, "National Survey on Americans as Healthcare Consumers: An Update on the Role of Quality Information," in *2002 AHA Environmental Assessment.* For a differential analysis of trust among Hispanic and African American patients, see L. E. Boulware et al., "Race and Trust in the Health Care System," *Public Health Reports* 118 (Jul–Aug 2003): 358–365.

14. Center for Studying Health System Change, *Who Do You Trust? Americans' Perspectives on Healthcare 1997–2001* (Washington, D.C.: Author, 2002). Even among those who fully participate in the healthcare system, surveys find a disparity of trust and satisfaction that falls along racial, ethnic, and economic lines. See S. E. Woods et al., "The Influence of Ethnicity on Patient Satisfaction," *Ethnicity & Health* 10 (2005): 235–242; L. S. Hicks et al., "Is Hospital Service Associated with Racial and Ethnic Disparities in Experiences with Hospital Care?" *American Journal of Medicine* 118 (2005): 529–535; and, F. M. Chen, "Patients' Beliefs About Racism, Preferences for Physician Race, and Satisfaction with Care," *Annals of Family Medicine* 3 (2005): 138–143.

15. Center for Studying Health System Change, *Who Do You Trust?* General patient trust in their own doctor also extends to the specialists who treat them and is higher if they have some role in selecting their provider. See Nancy L. Keating et al., "Patient Characteristics and Experiences Associated with Trust in Specialist Physicians," *Archives of Internal Medicine* 164 (2004): 1015–1020; David Mechanic, "In My Chosen Doctor I Trust," *British Medical Journal* 329 (2004): 1418–1419; and R. Balkrishnan et al., "Trust in Insurers and Access to Physicians: Associated Enrollee Behaviors and Changes over Time," *Health Services Research* 39 (2004): 813–823.

16. Harris Interactive Survey 2005, reported in "Public Attitudes to Hospitals, Pharmaceuticals and Managed Care Companies Improve Significantly," *Harris Interactive Healthcare News* (May 11, 2005.) 5 (4): 1.

17. See Boston Women's Health Book Collective, *Our Bodies, Ourselves,* 2nd edition (New York: Simon & Schuster, 1976). More recent editions are available as well.

18. Patients' trust in insurers and physicians is directly proportional to their sense of gatekeeping efforts among providers. See Marie C. Reed and Sally Trude, "Who Do You Trust? American Perspectives on Health Care, 1997–2001," *Center for Health System Change Tracking Report* no. 3 (Aug 2002): 1–4; Rajesh Balkrishnan et al., "Trust in Insurers"; and Jennifer S. Haas et al., "Is the Prevalence of Gatekeeping in a Community Associated with Individual Trust in Medical Care?" *Medical Care* 41 (2003): 660–668.

19. Mark Schlesinger, Shannon Mitchell, and Bradford H. Gray, "Public Expectations of Nonprofit and For-Profit Ownership in American Medicine: Clarifications and Implications," *Health Affairs* 23 (2004): 181–192; and Melissa M. Ahern and Michael S. Hendryx, "Social Capital and Trust in Providers," *Social Science & Medicine* 57 (2003): 1195–1203.

20. Linda H. Aiken, Sean P. Clarke, Douglas M. Sloane, Julie Sochalski, and Jeffrey H. Silber, "Hospital Nurse Staffing and Patient Mortality, Nurse Burnout, and Job Dissatisfaction," *Journal of the American Medical Association* 288 (2002): 1987–1993.

21. See the discussion in the chapter by Lucian Leape in this volume.

22. Barbara Starfield, "Is U.S. Health Really the Best in the World?" *The Journal of the American Medical Association* 284 (2000): 483–485.

23. A discussion of the chain e-mail and its various interpretations and critiques can be viewed at http://www.breakthechain.org/exclusives/drguns.html (accessed August 16, 2005).

24. J. Turow and R. Gans, *As Seen on TV: Health Policy Issues in TV's Medical Dramas,* Report to the Kaiser Family Foundation, July 2002. Available: http://www.kff.org/entmedia/John_Q_Report.pdf (accessed September 13, 2005). Curiously, in this climate many non-HMO enrollees mistakenly believe that they are covered by HMOs and therefore cultivate a more suspicious perception of their insurers. See J. D. Reschovsky, J. L. Hargraves, and A. F. Smith, "Consumer Beliefs and Health Plan Performance: It's Not Whether You Are in an HMO but Whether You Think You Are," *Journal of Health Politics, Policy and Law* 27 (2002): 353–377.

25. Kaiser Family Foundation, "Television Hospital Dramas Often Draw on Public Policy Debated for Story Lines, Study Says," *Daily Health Policy Report: Media and Society,* July 17, 2002. Available: http://www.kaisernetwork.org/daily_reports/rep_index.cfm?hint=3&DR_ID=12370 (accessed September 13, 2005).

26. "Response to the Movie John Q.," survey released at the Kaiser Family Foundation forum "John Q Goes to Washington: Health Policy Issues in Popular Culture," July 16, 2002, Washington, D.C.

27. David Mechanic argues that HMOs have been the target of misguided criticism generated by unfavorable media portrayals and sustained by the unrealistic expectations of patients. See David Mechanic, "Targeting HMOs: Stalemate in the U.S. Health Care Debate?" *Contexts* 3 (Spring 2004): 27–33.

28. *Wall Street Journal,* December 18, 2002, p. 1.

29. Walter C. Willett, *Eat, Drink, and Be Healthy: The Harvard Medical School Guide to Healthy Eating* (New York: Simon & Schuster, 2001), 28.

30. Other commentators have also noted multiple consequences of declining trust. See Donald Berwick, "The Importance and Paucity of Trust in Today's Health Care System," *Trustee* 58 (April 2005): 32–34.

31. Kaiser-Harvard National Survey of Americans' Views on Managed Care 1997, reported in "Is There A Managed Care 'Backlash'? Most Americans Give Their Own Health Plan a Good Grade, but Have Concerns about Key Aspects of Managed Care," November 5, 1997. Available: http://www.kff.org (accessed September 21, 2005).

32. According to Weiss, 2 million Medicare patients were "dumped" 1998–2000. "Medicare HMO Fiasco: Few Options Available for the Nearly One Million Seniors to Be Dropped from HMOs by Year-End," November 8, 2000, Weiss Ratings Inc. Available: http://www.weissratings.com/news/Ins_Medigap/20001108medigap.htm (accessed November 15, 2004).

33. See for example Felicia Trachtenberg et al., "How Patients' Trust Relates to Their Involvement in Medical Care," *Journal of Family Practice* 54 (2005): 344–352; Dana G. Safran et al., "Linking Primary Care Performance to Outcomes of Care," *Journal of Family Practice* 47 (1998): 213–220.

34. Terese Hudson Thrall, "New Nurse-Staffing Rules Present Big Challenge: Treat Patients or Violate the Law," *Hospitals & Health Networks* (January 2004): 24. Available: http://www.lexisnexis.com (accessed September 16, 2005).

35. This devotion to consistently high customer services is seen in the Mayo Clinic's efforts to build its brand. See Leonard L Berry and Neeli Bendapudi, "Clueing in Customers," *Harvard Business Review* 81, no. 2 (2003): 100–106, 126.

36. R. S. Tedlow and W. K. Smith, "James Burke: A Career in American Business (B)," Harvard Business School Case #9–390–030 (Boston: Harvard Business School, 1989).

37. For a discussion on the potential of "power brands" in healthcare, see Michael Petromilli and Dorothy Michalczyk, "Your Most Valuable Asset: Increasing the Value of Your Hospital through Its Brand," *Marketing Health Services* 19, no. 2 (1999): 4–9.

2

Why Americans Don't Trust the Government and Don't Trust Healthcare

ROBERT J. BLENDON

Surely a question on the minds of virtually every healthcare provider and administrator today must be what did we do to deserve this? *This,* of course, refers to the rapid drop in Americans' expressed confidence—trust—in the people running the medical system. In 1966, 73 percent of poll respondents said they felt "a great deal" of confidence in medicine. That number then began a long-term decline and in 1991 hit an all-time low of 20 percent. By 2004, it had climbed a little, to 32 percent (Figure 2.1). Still, a 32 percent confidence level is not a number calculated to help healthcare providers sleep comfortably at night.

At first glance, it is not entirely clear why trust should have declined so much and so rapidly. Certainly, American healthcare has its failings. But the record over the last 35 years is mostly one of improvement, not decline. New drugs and technologies preserve and prolong lives that would have been lost in the 1960s. Life expectancy at birth has increased roughly seven years—about 10 percent—since 1966.[1] Patients seeking advanced care fly to leading U.S. medical centers from all over the world. Moreover, the majority of Americans continue to express high levels of trust in their personal physicians. In 2002, for example, 81 percent said that they trusted their doctor to do the right thing for their medical care "just about always" or "most of the time."[2]

So why the drop? As it happens, this phenomenon is now fairly well understood. The explanation may be easier to grasp if we begin not with the decline in trust of the healthcare industry but with the similar decline in Americans' trust in government. The parallels are instructive.

Government: The Dynamics of Distrust

As Harvard historian Ernest R. May reminds us, people who were deeply distrustful of government founded the United States.[3] This lack of trust lives on. In

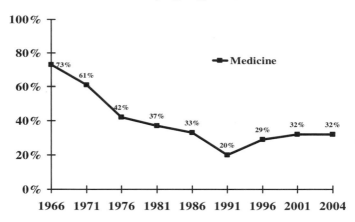

Figure 2.1. Public confidence in medicine

Source: Data from Harris Interactive Polls, 1966–2004. Available: http://www.harrisinteractive
.com/harris_poll/index.asp?PID=447 (accessed April 19, 2006).

a 1998 poll, for instance, some 56 percent of Americans said that they basically
distrusted government, a number exceeded among Western nations only by
France (59 percent).[4] More specific indicators of trust have declined markedly
over the past four decades. In the early 1960s, for example, roughly three-quarters
of Americans said they trusted the federal government to do the right thing "always" or "most of the time." By 1992 this number had plummeted to roughly one-
quarter. And though it rose abruptly in the wake of September 11, 2001, it has
since dropped again (Figure 2.2).

The trend of decline, with its occasional upward and downward turns, can be
plotted against historical events. When we do this we find two patterns of correspondence. The first might be called major government failures in performance,
and it illustrates a fundamental truth about trust: People judge government not by
what any individual agency does but by their perception of how things are going
overall. Are there big problems? Does the public believe that government leaders
are acting effectively to solve those problems? In the mid-to-late 1960s and early
1970s, the nation's biggest single problem in most Americans' minds was the Vietnam War, and nearly everyone thought the government should be doing something
different from what it was doing. There were other problems on people's minds as
well. The economy in the 1970s was in serious difficulty, plagued by sluggish
growth and high inflation. The two energy crises in 1973 and 1979 created hard-
ship and uncertainty for millions of Americans, and the government seemed ineffective in dealing with them, just as it seemed ineffective in dealing with the
1979–1980 U.S. hostage crisis in Iran. Another factor in the decline of trust,
it turns out, was the rising crime rate during the 1970s. It hardly mattered that
crime prevention in the United States is not a major responsibility of the federal

government; people simply felt that "if the government can't protect me from violent crime, then I don't have confidence in the government." The condemnation extended to all levels.

A second pattern of correspondence between the graph and national events lies in scandals, which have a galvanizing effect on people's levels of trust. The Watergate scandal contributed significantly to the decline in trust during the 1970s. The Iran-Contra scandal helped undermine the upward blip of trust enjoyed by the Reagan administration during the 1980s. The Whitewater and Lewinsky scandals helped keep trust levels relatively low during the Clinton administration. What is curious about scandals, of course, is that corruption was arguably much more widespread in the past. The difference today is that the media can (and do) run virtually nonstop coverage of scandals. People can see pictures—over and over again—of a congressman taking a bribe or of a president's associate going to jail. That feeds the perception that corruption is growing worse every day, and indeed that it may be at its worst point ever.

A third factor affecting the decline in trust is harder to pin down and is discussed at greater length by Pippa Norris (see chapter 3). There has been a cultural change in industrialized countries over the last three or four decades. The story runs essentially as follows. When people are better educated and better off economically, they feel less threatened and insecure. The less they feel threatened and insecure, the less they are likely to trust figures of authority. The correlation between threat and trust can be seen most starkly in wartime. The highest presidential job-approval ratings ever recorded were in early 1942, right after the attack on Pearl Harbor. And immediately after the attack on the World Trade Towers on September 11, 2001, the level of trust (see Figure 2.2) more than doubled, from 30

Percent saying "always/most of time"

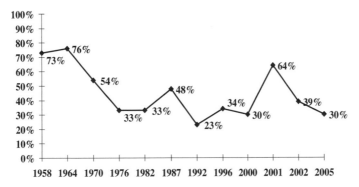

Figure 2.2. Trust in the federal government to do the right thing

Source: Data from American National Election Studies, "Trust the Government,1958–1982," University of Michigan. Available: http://www.umich.edu/~nes/nesguide/toptable/tab5a_1.htm (accessed April 19, 2006); ABC News and *Washington Post* Polls (1987–2002) and Gallup Poll (2005) available from the Roper Center for Public Opinion Research, Storrs, Connecticut.

percent to 64 percent. When people feel insecure, they need to believe in an authority figure. But as feelings of security return, the level of trust declines (witness the drop in trust after September 11). And over time, trust in government is lower among people who are better educated and better off.

Interestingly, trust in the government is not related to personal experience with government. Virtually every study reveals this somewhat counterintuitive fact. Almost no one witnesses a government official taking a bribe. Only a tiny minority of citizens are directly affected by perceived government ineptitude; even in an economic downturn, only a few people out of every hundred lose their jobs. Where trust is concerned, perceptions are important, and the media creates and nurtures perceptions. We hear over and over again about all the people who do lose their jobs in a recession. We see reports of malfeasance in high places repeatedly. We are afraid to walk in our neighborhoods not because we personally have been attacked or because we know someone who was, but because the media tells us that people are being attacked in other neighborhoods like ours. This lesson is worth bearing in mind as we shift gears and look at healthcare and confront the question posed at the beginning of this chapter: What did we do to deserve this?

Trust in the federal government can matter for healthcare. Look again at Figure 2.2, which shows the level of public trust in the federal government to do the right thing. The enactment of Medicare happened when trust was high, during the mid-1960s. Trust hit rock-bottom in 1992, as the last great healthcare reform debate began. When Hillary Clinton's task force issued its 1,700-page proposal, it was essentially dead on arrival.

Lack of Trust in Healthcare

In general, the dynamics of declining trust in healthcare correspond very closely to the dynamics of declining trust in government. Ever since the 1970s, for example, polls have shown that Americans have worried most about two healthcare issues. One is continually rising costs. The other is the large number of people who remain uninsured.[5] These are perceived as the major problems of healthcare. As we have seen from the analysis of trust in government, trust declines when people believe that leaders are not effectively addressing major issues.

The effect of scandals is similar as well. What kind of scandals plague healthcare? One sort—unfortunately recurrent and often given wide play in the media—is the medical error. A doctor or a hospital makes a mistake, and a patient dies. A second sort of scandal is known in the medical world as the "impaired physician," but is usually referred to as problem doctors. These are doctors with drug or alcohol problems, or problems with mental illness, who do terrible things to patients. A third sort of scandal is the doctor or hospital found to be bilking insurance companies or Medicare, fattening his or her own purse at the expense of premium payers or taxpayers.

The exposure of most scandals follows a familiar pattern. A lawyer or journalist pursues an alleged wrongdoer. When the story breaks, it often turns out that the doctor in question has been in and out of professional reviews for years, but his or her license was never suspended and no action was taken. At worst, an offending doctor might have been put on temporary suspension or sent to another hospital. It often seems from press accounts that the problem doctor's colleagues feel nothing but empathy for them, while ignoring the legitimate complaints of the abused patients or the payers from whom they embezzled money. It also may appear that the leadership of the profession is doing nothing to address such problems. The public heard in the late 1990s the news of a deal (later rescinded) in which the American Medical Association (AMA) agreed to endorse Sunbeam products in return for a percentage of every Sunbeam item sold. It has not heard the news of a major, new AMA campaign to deal with inept or pernicious doctors.

No one should underestimate the importance of the leadership's reaction to scandals. For instance, among the 10 institutions whose trust levels have been tracked by opinion polls in the last 30 years, the only one that actually rose in the public's estimation was the military. Part of that increase in trust, no doubt, reflects the military's low starting point—an effect of the unpopular Vietnam War—and the boost it enjoyed from the nearly bloodless military action in Granada and later from the 1991 Gulf War. But during this era, the leaders of the military also placed a great deal of emphasis on developing and enforcing a code of ethics. People began to feel that military leadership stood for something, and that leaders were trying to bring ethical behavior to the entire institution. They did not feel the same about the leadership of the medical profession or indeed about the leadership of most other institutions.

However, people do not mistrust their personal physicians. Individual doctors enjoy the 81 percent approval rating mentioned above, and some 77 percent of poll respondents say they would trust their physician to tell them if a mistake were made in their treatment.[6] These are both extraordinarily high numbers. Asked if they trust physicians to make the right decisions about their healthcare, 43 percent of poll respondents say they have a great deal of confidence that physicians will do so, while only 12 percent say they have little or no confidence (Figure 2.3).

Institutions: The Pattern of Decline

The parallels between healthcare and other sectors of society are even stronger when we move from the individual practitioner to the institutional and organizational level. Research about the decline of trust in institutions and organizations reveals a distinct pattern in many different fields of endeavor. The bare bones of the pattern look like this:

1. Something happens. Some members of an industry do something that dramatically raises the public's fears about their personal safety or that seems outrageously and financially exploitative.
2. Such events are dramatic, and they must seriously challenge public values, the values by which people live.

Percent saying "a great deal"

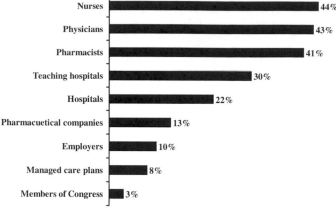

Figure 2.3. Trust in various groups to make the right decision about your health care
Source: Data from Harris Interactive Poll (New York: Harris Interactive, March 2002).

3. These events provoke a sharp decline in trust, even if consumer satisfaction with the industry in question is otherwise high.
4. Trust declines, even though very few people have any direct negative experience with the industry.

The pattern is illustrated below with examples from various institutions, then examined as it applies to healthcare.

The Catholic Church

Consider the recent revelations concerning the abuse of youngsters by Catholic priests. Surveys show that the majority of Catholics have no experience with abuse by priests. Surveys also show that most people found their last experience at church religiously rewarding, and that they have a great deal of respect for their priests. Nonetheless, many Catholics have lost their trust in the institution as a whole, because a small number of cases challenge the fundamental values that the church represents, and because church leaders apparently took no decisive action to end the abuse. Support for the church leadership has plummeted, even though the scandal has nothing to do with average Catholics' experiences or relationships with their priests.

Accounting

It is much the same with the accounting profession. Most Americans who have accountants do not find them shredding documents in their offices. They actually think that accountants are reliable people. When accounting clients are asked "How satisfied are you with the last visit to your accountant?" their responses are generally positive. But it is not hard to imagine how trust in the accounting profession has declined in the wake of the corporate scandals of recent years. The accounting firms serving two of the largest companies in the world destroyed information and helped plunge their clients into bankruptcy. The firms were indirectly responsible for the loss of tens of thousands of jobs and hundreds of billions of dollars in market value. It was an abuse that threatened the fundamental values of the market economy.

Banking

Track the public's attitudes toward an institution over time and you can see very clearly both the causes and the results of a rapid decline in trust; you can also understand something about what might be called the epidemiology of scandals. The story of banking in the late 20th century depicts this dynamic. In the 1970s and 1980s, only about one-fourth of poll respondents said there was a need for more government regulation of banking (Figure 2.4). In 1991, that trust suddenly plummeted, and more than 50 percent of poll respondents favored more government regulation. What happened in the interim, of course, was the savings and loan scandal, in which several savings and loan institutions were bailed out with taxpayers' dollars.

The interesting thing about this example is that 75 percent of Americans had no money in a savings and loan, and only two states out of 50 had no protection

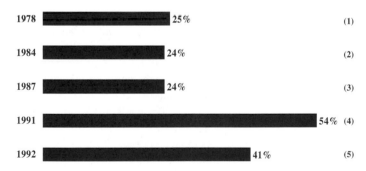

Percent saying "needs more"

1978	25%	(1)
1984	24%	(2)
1987	24%	(3)
1991	54%	(4)
1992	41%	(5)

Figure 2.4. Public view of whether there is a need for more government regulation of banking

Source: Data from (1) Yankelovich, Skelly & White/American Council of Life Insurance Poll, 1978; (2) Roper Report Poll, 1984; (3) Roper Report Poll, 1987; (4) Los Angeles Times Poll, 1991; (5) Wirthlin Group Poll, 1992. Available from the Roper Center for Public Opinion Research, Storrs, Connecticut.

for savings and loan depositors. Epidemiologically speaking, this was a minor, contained outbreak. But that was not how the public perceived it. In effect, people said, "I don't have any money in a savings and loan, but I *never* want to walk into a bank and have them tell me my money's gone." The banks, of course, held a different view. Commercial banks argued that they were not savings and loans and should not be tarred with the same brush. They argued further that their customers were highly satisfied with their services; indeed, poll results showed only a minor decline in customer satisfaction with banks from the 1980s to the early 1990s.[7] But it didn't matter. Consumers suddenly were crying for banks to be regulated. A few people had stolen a significant amount of money; the institutions involved had tried to cover it up; and Congress was at first unwilling to address the problem. That is exactly what leads to an abrupt decline in trust.

Airlines

This, too, is an industry where trust levels changed markedly over time. In 1987, 55 percent of the public believed that airlines needed more government regulation; in 1996 the level was up to 78 percent. In 1995, only 39 percent believed that current regulations were "fair" or "poor"; in 1996 that number had jumped to 54 percent. What happened in between can be summarized easily: the tragic, dramatic, and well-publicized crash of a ValuJet airliner in Florida in May 1996.

Again, the epidemiology is instructive. In 1987 there were six million commercial flights and seven accidents. In 1996 there were eight million flights and only five accidents. Theoretically, travelers should have been feeling better about air safety. As for customer satisfaction, in 1987 there were 11,000 complaints, while in 1996 there were about 6,000. That trend line, too, was in the direction of greater trust. But once more, none of this mattered. Suddenly, the downed airliner was on the front pages of newspapers across the country. Suddenly investigators were reporting that ValuJet had a penny-pinching culture that may have compromised safety. The public concluded that airlines could not be trusted to protect their lives and that government regulations had been ineffective. Period.

The examples could go on and on. For instance, most Americans do not get their power from nuclear power plants; most don't even live within 500 miles of one. Those who do get nuclear-generated power pronounce themselves satisfied: the electricity works, and the price is reasonable. But public support for stricter regulation of nuclear power plants jumped after the Three Mile Island incident in June 1976 and jumped again after the Chernobyl incident in April 1986. In the latter case, the unimportance of personal experience could hardly be clearer. Chernobyl is many thousands of miles away from America. The plant operated under a corrupt and dying regime. But Americans responded to the incident by demanding stricter regulation of *American* nuclear plants. In effect, the public declared that anything remotely resembling Chernobyl was utterly unacceptable. And people suddenly had less confidence that the nuclear industry in America could be trusted to prevent such a disaster.

Lessons for Healthcare

In looking at the opening question for healthcare—What did we do to deserve this?—I want to focus on managed care, which is perhaps the most problematic area of the healthcare system from a trust perspective. If managed care executives look only at Americans' ratings of experience with their current health plan, they might easily conclude that everything is copacetic. In one recent poll, for example, some 68 percent of the public rated their experience as "excellent" or "good," with only a tiny minority saying it was "poor" or "failing." And yet when the public's views on the managed care industry are rated over time, the percent saying it is doing a good job for consumers dropped from 51 percent in 1997 to 29 percent in 2001, and remained at 30 percent in 2004.[8] This is a sharp decline in trust.

The reason for the decline follows the same pattern as the other institutions. For example, in 1997 a young woman died from breast cancer and her father sued her HMO, charging that they had denied her access to the latest care throughout her illness. The story was reported in the *Boston Globe* and other newspapers. Such an event is not likely to be unique, but it is likely to be rare. The vast majority of HMO plan members are highly unlikely to be involved in a similar experience.

But the experience of other industries illuminates how people react to this kind of event. Just as nobody wants to feel that an airline or a nuclear power plant might compromise their safety, nobody wants to belong to a health plan that might needlessly cost them their life. That is the fundamental value here: People assume that nobody who ran a health plan would ever do that to them. They wouldn't let anybody die. But now somebody did die, and suddenly the thought occurs to people across America that their plan, a plan run by the kind of individuals they knew in high school or college, could make a decision that allowed somebody to die. Consider a poll that asked respondents, in effect, whether they believed the headline. The statement was "A family says their HMO held back on their child's cancer treatment," and people were asked to say how often they thought that actually happened. Twenty-six percent of respondents said "often." Another 40 percent said "sometimes."[9] Put bluntly, two-thirds of Americans felt that managed care plans might permit people to die for lack of care.

This is the equivalent of the Catholic priest issue: In America, that behavior is unacceptable. People who run health plans cannot put people's lives at risk. Asked if health plans should pay for treatment even if it costs a million dollars per life, nearly two-thirds of Americans responded that they should.[10] That view affects trust in the entire industry, and it has little or nothing to do with whether any individual reacted positively to his or her last experience with a health plan.

Another fair question might be "so what?" Should a managed care plan or any other healthcare organization really be concerned about a decline in trust, if its customers are having satisfactory experiences? After all, a devil's advocate might argue, R. J. Reynolds and the other tobacco companies have been at the bottom of the trust scale for decades, yet they have continued to prosper. Is healthcare so different? In fact, a lack of trust has three major effects on an industry, all delete-rious. Avoiding them is surely one obligation of any executive who takes a view longer than the next quarter's financial results.

The first—an effect that can take 15 or 20 years before it is felt—is jury trials. It turns out that if a distrusted industry loses a major trial, juries tend to decide that they will make up for everything that has gone wrong in the previous 20 years. When the tobacco awards began to mount up, the juries were effectively saying "We don't want to fine these companies, we want to punish them. We want to put them out of business." It was much the same with asbestos, the effects of which the industry covered up for years. When the health problems finally caught up with the companies, the jury settlements were unbelievable. In this case, the juries did put the industry out of business.

From managed care's perspective, what is worrisome is not the average law-suit. Most can be successfully fought or settled. The real concern is the block-buster lawsuit, that plays off a well-publicized case, like the suit brought by the father of the woman who died of breast cancer. In time, some such suit will come to trial, and the industry will lose when the jury decides to punish them for their alleged misdeeds. The punishment could be enormous.

The second effect is increased government regulation. If an industry suffers from a lack of trust, the public will want the government to regulate it. People were willing to buy unsafe cars for years, but the revelations about auto safety led to a fundamental lack of trust in the industry and a cry for greater regulation. These cries eventually fell on receptive ears in Congress. No politician wants to stand up in the legislature and propose to regulate an industry that the public trusts, but when the public loses confidence in an industry, politicians smell blood. There have been dozens of bills in government legislatures to regulate managed care organizations more closely. This should come as no surprise to anyone who understands the dynamics of trust.

Finally, the trust issue affects the environment people work in. If you work in managed care, for instance, are you proud to tell your children and your neighbors what you do? Do you dread reading the paper, or looking at the editorial cartoons, or even watching television because you fear that your industry may be under at-tack? Health care institutions of all sorts once enjoyed a high reputation among the public, a reputation that has come under attack in recent years. It would be nice for those who work in the industry to get the reputation back.

Getting it back is not magic. It involves leadership that does not ignore major problems, that reacts firmly and ethically to scandals the minute they break and does not try to cover them up, and that understands how the consequences of seemingly small decisions can loom large. On a personal note, I have been a re-viewer for a number of television news magazines. The producers of one program were doing segments on managed care, and they would send me dramatic cases about somebody who had been denied care for a serious illness. I understood that the cases weren't representative; that they were rare; and that they did not repre-sent managed care fairly. But again, it didn't matter. When I looked at those cases, every value that I treasure, every value that holds a society together, seemed to be threatened by the decisions to deny benefits to those people. And when the shows ran over and over again, viewers sat at home and said, "This can't be happening. People can't allow this to happen." The trust meter for managed care took another plunge.

The tragedy is that, had leaders understood the importance of these decisions and not relegated them to some midlevel manager who was just trying to do a job, trust might have been maintained, even increased. But leaders are often short-sighted: They fail to take the long view and to take the steps necessary to build trust. *That* is what they have done to deserve the decline in trust over the past few decades.

Notes

1. U.S. Census Bureau, *Historical Statistics of the United States, Colonial Times to 1970, Vol. 1* (Washington, D.C.: U.S. Government Printing Office, 1975), 55; and, U.S. Census Bureau, *Statistical Abstract of the United States, 2000* (Washington, D.C.: U.S. Government Printing Office, 2000), 84.

2. NPR/Kaiser Family Foundation/Kennedy School of Government, "National Survey on Health Care," (June 2002). Available: http://www.kff.org/kaiserpolls/loader.cfm?url=/commonspot/security/getfile.cfm&PageID=14064 (accessed June 14, 2005).

3. See Ernest R. May, "The Evolving Scope of Government," in *Why People Don't Trust Government,* ed. Joseph S. Nye et al. (Cambridge, Mass.: Harvard University Press, 1997), 21–55.

4. Pew Research Center for the People and the Press, "Deconstructing Distrust: How Americans View Government," February 1998. Available: http://people-press.org/dataarchive/ (accessed June 14, 2005).

5. Recent public concerns about healthcare are described in Robert J. Blendon et al., "Health Care in the 2004 Presidential Election," *New England Journal of Medicine* 351 (2004): 1314–1323.

6. NPR/Kaiser Family Foundation/Kennedy School of Government, "National Survey on Health Care."

7. Gallup/American Society for Quality Control Polls. (Storrs, Conn.: Roper Center for Public Opinion Research, July 1985, June 1988, June 1991).

8. Harris Interactive Polls, 1997–2004. Data summarized in "Supermarkets, Food Companies, Airlines, Computers and Banks Top the List of Industries Doing a Good Job for Their Consumers," *The Harris Poll*, no. 38, May 28, 2004. Available: http://www.harrisinteractive.com/harris_poll/index.asp?PID=467 (accessed August 19, 2005).

9. Robert J. Blendon, Mollyann Brodie, John M. Benson, Drew E. Altman, Larry Levitt, Tina Hoff, and Larry Hugick, "Understanding the Managed Care Backlash." *Health Affairs*, 1998, 17(4):80–94. For additional data on public concerns over health plans' influence on medical decision making, see Marie C. Reed and Sally Trude, "Who Do You Trust? Americans' Perspectives on Health Care, 1997–2001," *HSC Tracking Report*, no. 3 (Aug. 2002).

10. Robert J. Blendon et al., "Who Has the Best Health Care System? A Second Look," *Health Affairs* 14, no. 4 (1995): 220–230.

3

Skeptical Patients: Performance, Social Capital, and Culture

PIPPA NORRIS

Medicine faces a major challenge today. As my colleague Robert J. Blendon shows in chapter 2, public trust and confidence in the healthcare profession in America, while remaining high in comparison with many similar institutions, has been steadily eroding since the mid-1960s.

The concept of trust is understood here as *the expectation that others will act in one's interest,* that is, A trusts B to do X. It can apply to particular individuals, to social groups, or to institutions like banks, airlines, or Congress. In medicine, trust is commonly thought to play a vital role in patient-physician relations. Trusted doctors are those believed to act in the interest of their patients by providing competent advice, responsible treatment, and compassionate care that contributes effectively to patients' well being. Trust may facilitate patient-physician communications in ways that enhance diagnosis, treatment, and compliance. Moreover, a general erosion of confidence in medicine as an institution may gradually undermine the political legitimacy and scientific authority of the healthcare profession.

Three different schools of thought have sought to explain the decline of trust. *Institutional performance–based* accounts focus on specific organizational changes in the practice of healthcare in America, such as the increased size and centralization of health plans, the growth of managed care, the substantial budget that drug companies devote to advertising, and the impact of these developments on the patient-physician relationship. *Social capital* theories focus on the role of dense networks of associations generating social trust and institutional confidence. In particular, these theories look toward the strength of the face-to-face bonds between the family physician and their patients, the attenuation and weakening of these bonds by the professionalization of medicine, and the displacement of the general practitioner by the rise of expert specialists. In contrast, *cultural* accounts suggest that the growth of skeptical attitudes toward medicine reflects a more general process of value change in many modern societies. In this perspective, attitudes towards medicine form part of a broader challenge to traditional sources of professional authority; they reflect an erosion of faith in multiple private and public sector institutions, affecting doctors as well as religious, educational, corporate, political, and military leaders. The core explanation here focuses on changes in mass society, notably the growth of cognitive skills and the rise of a more critical public in postindustrial nations, rather than on the performance of institutions.

To examine these theories, evidence is drawn from trends in institutional confidence first monitored in Harris surveys during the mid-1960s and in the General Social Survey (GSS) conducted annually by the National Opinion Research Center (NORC) since the early 1970s. This study confirms that confidence in medicine has indeed eroded during the last three decades, but far from being sector-specific, the pattern reflects trends in many other comparable institutions in the private, nonprofit, and public sectors, including education, unions, organized religion, Congress and the Executive branch, the military, major companies, and the mass media. Social trust is associated with institutional confidence, but only weakly. The most plausible interpretation is that a long-term process of cultural change has altered the traditional patient-physician relationship in the United States as well as in other affluent postindustrial societies. The most convincing explanation lies in long-term changes in the mass public, such as rising cognitive levels and less deference toward authority, rather than in the delivery of healthcare per se or a puzzling failure of performance afflicting all major institutions in society. Moreover, the erosion of confidence in medicine is not confined to specific social sectors, such as African Americans, the poor, or those with health problems, instead it occurs fairly uniformly throughout all major groups in America.

This chapter first considers longstanding debates in the literature about the causes of growing mistrust of societal and political institutions, including the role of performance, social capital, and cultural shifts, which form the broader theoretical context for understanding confidence in medicine. Then evidence is examined for trends concerning confidence in 13 major institutions, including medicine, based on baseline figures from Harris surveys conducted in the mid-1960s with trends updated by the GSS every year from 1972 to 2000. The patterns of trust in medicine are broken down further by age and cohort analysis to examine the root causes of these developments. Finally, the chapter focuses on the factors that can help to explain trends in confidence in medicine across the pooled GSS sample, using multivariate models, including the standard social background variables of age, education, race, income, gender, and religiosity, as well as exposure to the mass media, the role of social trust, and the reported state of health. To place the trends in context, the study also considers alternative indicators of attitudes towards doctors and trusted information sources in health and medicine. The conclusion summarizes the results and considers alternative interpretations of their implications for the future of healthcare and patient-physician relations.

Theories of Trust and Confidence

In the last decade, we have witnessed a substantial revival of interest within sociology and philosophy in the role of trust as a public and private good.[1] What can explain a loss of public trust and confidence in medicine? At least three schools of thought attempt to explain this phenomenon: those that concentrate on institutional performance, those that emphasize social capital and trust, and those that focus on cultural shifts occurring across postindustrial societies.

The Institutional Performance Model

The first model focuses on the actual performance of institutions as the key to understanding citizens' confidence in them. Healthcare institutions that perform well are likely to elicit the confidence of citizens; those that perform badly or ineffectively generate feelings of distrust and low confidence. The general public, this model assumes, recognizes whether institutions are performing well or poorly and reacts accordingly.

This is a popular perspective. Many commentators, for example, have argued that changes in managed care have contributed toward growing skepticism toward medicine.[2] Hence, Illingworth suggests that developments in healthcare have compromised the ability of doctor-patient relations to generate trust; Illingworth blames in particular the rise of managed care, the increased size and centralization of healthcare plans, cost-containment mechanisms, increased regulatory interventions, and price competition.[3] As Emanuel and Dubler summarize this perspective, the ideal physician-patient relationship has been undermined by the expansion of managed healthcare, particularly by the limits on patients' choice of healthcare services; by productivity requirements that increase time pressures on healthcare professionals that can undermine communication; by disruptions in the continuity of care; and by increased conflict of interest due to salary schemes that reward physicians for not using medical services.[4] Mechanic emphasizes that the commercialization of medical care, conflict of interest, and the growth of managed healthcare have all challenged the extent to which patients see their doctors as competent, responsible, and caring, and hence how much they trust them; this situation has been compounded by mass media attention to medical uncertainty and error. Mechanic argues that trust is encouraged by patient choice, continuity of care, and consultancy time that allows opportunities for feedback, as well as by patient participation in medical decisions.[5] Institutions have responded to this concern with a variety of measures designed to restore trust, including eliciting patient feedback, providing more information for patients, improving staff training in interpersonal skills, instituting patient empowerment projects, and focusing on ethical issues.

The performance theory has three broad implications. First, given accurate sampling techniques, reliable research procedures, and sensible survey questions, responses to questionnaire items about institutional confidence are likely to be a good gauge of how well the healthcare system is actually performing. In other words, confidence questions are likely to provide an accurate thermometer of public life. Second, the theory suggests that if medical institutions earn little public esteem, the remedy for the situation lies in either lowering public expectations of performance (medical science can promise less) or in improving institutional effectiveness (healthcare professionals can deliver more).

Third, the model suggests that some may be more critical of healthcare performance than others. In particular we might expect that those in poor health, the less affluent, and ethnic minority groups might be more negative toward the introduction of managed care. Conversely, the model also suggests that there might be little differentiation across society, if the general public has become more critical of healthcare services. This is because confidence in medical institutions is the product of their overall performance in much the same way that perception of the trustworthiness of others and willingness to trust them are based on the experience of how others behave. Moreover, medical performance affects individuals regardless of their particular social type. Not all citizens are equally affected by healthcare, but systemic medical problems such as prohibitive prescription costs, excessive delays for basic treatment, and dramatic health scares such as major failures of food safety have an impact on all citizens to a greater or lesser extent. This explains why trust and distrust in medicine tend to be more or less randomly distributed among people with different characteristics, such as education, income, religion, age, or gender.

The institutional performance model thus does not predict a strong relationship between social characteristics and confidence in institutions. On the contrary, it leads us to expect that changes in trust in medicine will vary according to the actual or perceived institutional performance of healthcare. The most appropriate evidence examines trends in confidence among different institutions. If confidence declines consistently and steadily across all major social institutions—such as schools *and* churches, banks *and* trade unions, Congress *and* the Executive branch—as well as medicine, then, unless we assume a sudden puzzling crisis in the performance of all these pillars of society, there must be something going on beyond how healthcare institutions perform.

The Social Capital Model

Posing an alternative to the performance model, some social theorists hold that the ability to trust others and sustain cooperative relations is the product of socialization and social experiences, especially those found in the sorts of voluntary associations that bring different social types together to achieve a common goal. The theory originates with Alexis de Tocqueville and John Stuart Mill, both of whom emphasized the importance of voluntary associations and social engagement as training grounds for democracy. Many contemporary writers pursue the same theme, discussing society's ability to inculcate "habits of the heart" such as trust, reciprocity, and cooperation, emphasizing the importance of civil society in generating cooperative social relations, or focusing on trust or civic culture as a basis for stable and peaceful democracy. A revival of interest in this idea has been fueled in no small measure by Putnam's work on social capital, civic engagement, and good governance, as well as by general concern about the consequences of an erosion of trust and confidence in many major societal and governmental institutions. [6] Much of this work has focused on the United States, but a growing literature has sought to compare whether similar trends are evident in postindustrial societies elsewhere.

The social and cultural model essentially argues that individual life situations and experiences—especially higher education, participation in a community with a cooperative culture, and involvement in voluntary activities—create social trust and cooperation, civic-mindedness, and reciprocity between individuals. This in turn helps create strong, effective, and successful social organizations and institutions, including community groups and social institutions in which people can invest their confidence. Such organizations and institutions in turn help build trust, cooperation, and reciprocity, as well as confidence in other institutions. In short, there is a direct and mutually reinforcing relationship between the types of people who express trust and confidence on the one hand and strong and effective social organizations and institutions on the other. If this is true, we would expect to find that people who express attitudes of trust toward medicine are likely to be well integrated into voluntary associations and other forms of cooperative social activity and to display high social trust.[7] Moreover, a trusting physician-patient relationship can be expected to develop with repeated face-to-face encounters over a sustained period of time, building up long-term, deep relationships. The ideal model here in healthcare is the general practitioner, who is familiar to family, neighbors, and friends in the local community and who deals with illnesses and life-altering events from birth to death.[8] This association can be tested only in a limited manner here with the available data, but we can examine the relationship between social trust and institutional confidence.[9]

Cultural Shifts and Modernization Theory

A third set of explanations—cultural explanations based on modernization theory—suggest that value change in postindustrial societies has encouraged the development of a more critical public who question all traditional sources of authority, whether religious, scientific, or moral. Modernization theories suggest that economic, cultural, and political changes go together in coherent ways, so that industrialization brings broadly similar trajectories, even if situation-specific factors make it impossible to predict exactly what will happen in a given society: certain changes become increasingly likely to occur, but the changes are probabilistic, not deterministic. Modernization theories originated in the work of Karl Marx, Max Weber, and Emile Durkheim. These ideas were revived and popularized in the late 1950s and early 1960s by Seymour Martin Lipset, Daniel Lerner, Walt Rostow, and Karl Deutsch. Recently, they have been developed most fully in the work of Ronald Inglehart.[10]

In poorer agrarian societies, Inglehart suggests, people live with high levels of insecurity and so tend to develop cultures mistrustful of rapid change. These agrarian cultures emphasize the values of traditional authority and strong leadership, inherited social status, and communal ties and obligations, backed up by social sanctions and norms derived from religious authorities. The rise of capitalism and the Industrial Revolution brought challenges to traditional values in the form of a worldview that encouraged achievement rather than ascribed status, individualism rather than community, innovation instead of continuity with tradition, and increasingly secular and scientific rather than religious social beliefs. During the post–World War II decades, Inglehart argues, postindustrial societies have gradually experienced a major shift in their basic cultural attitudes due to the modernization process. They attained unprecedented levels of prosperity and economic security, with rising standards of living fueled by generally steady economic growth. The development of postmaterialist values among the younger generation has been marked by a gradual decline in support for traditional sources of authority, including representative government and established, hierarchical institutions such as the army, police, and church. Faith in science and medicine has also been influenced by these developments, as demonstrated by the growth of alternative medicine and homeopathic remedies. Higher levels of education, fueling greater cognitive skills, increased access to information via the mass media, and long-term generational shifts are the root causes of these developments. The implication of value change is that, if correct, the erosion of faith in societal institutions is a process that is difficult if not impossible to reverse in affluent nations. Certain fluctuations can be expected due to "period-effects"—for example, blips upward or downward following eras of economic boom or bust—but the general trend should be a slow, steady secular erosion of faith evident across all major societal and governing institutions, not confined to particular sectors such as healthcare.

Trends in Institutional Trust

There are many alternative measures gauging attitudes toward healthcare professionals and confidence in medicine. A detailed multi-item Trust in Physician Scale has been developed with high consistency and reliability, but although it is valuable, we need simpler indicators to gauge trends over time.[11] This study draws on the baseline Harris surveys that were first fielded in 1966 and then the series of annual General Social Surveys conducted by NORC since 1973, using a representative sample of the adult population. These surveys used the following item:

> *I am going to name some institutions in this country. As far as the people running these institutions are concerned, would you say you have a great deal of confidence, only some confidence, or hardly any confidence at all in them?*

Almost three-quarters of the public (71 percent) expressed confidence in medicine in the 1966 Harris survey; medicine was the most highly rated institution in the comparison, coming in ahead of the military, education, and the Supreme Court. The 1973 NORC survey revealed a sharp fall across all institutions, with confidence in medicine down to a bare majority of the public (55 percent). Of course, some of the decline may be due to fieldwork and sampling differences between the two organizations, but previous detailed analysis by Lipset and Schneider suggests that there was a real shift during this era, one that was closely associated with the "hot-button" politics of these tumultuous years in American life, including the generational divisions over the Vietnam War, the civil rights movement, racial conflict, and the rise of new social movements.[12] In 1973, medicine was still the most highly ranked institution in the comparison, followed by science, education, and religion, and confidence remained relatively high until 1980. Then it began to slip. By 2000, 44 percent expressed a great deal of confidence in medicine, just behind science and ahead of the military. A comparison in the change across all institutions where we have the full time-series data suggests that confidence in education has slipped more, but the loss of faith in medicine is roughly similar to that experienced in Congress and major companies (prior to the Enron debacle). The evidence suggests that far from being sui generis, trust and confidence in medicine has experienced similar erosion to that found in other major institutions in American life, both public and private.

Age and Cohort Analysis

To examine this further, confidence in medicine was broken down for each decade by age group and by cohort of birth. The results suggest that from the 1970s to the 1990s confidence in medicine has correlated inversely with age. The young have always had more confidence in medicine than the old, possibly because they have been less dependent on it. The association between age and confidence has stayed about the same throughout the period, but may have weakened very slightly in the 1990s. However, the level of confidence in medicine fell between the 1970s and the 1990s among the public as a whole and in all age categories. The largest declines in confidence are among the middle age categories—the 35- to 64-year-olds. This reflects a "cohort" effect: the younger the cohort in the 1970s, the steeper the decline. This suggests that possibly there has been a sharper fall in confidence in all institutions among the 1970s young cohort, as a post-Vietnam, post-Watergate phenomenon, which has affected attitudes to medicine along with everything else.

Explaining Confidence in Medicine

Social Groups

If the performance explanation is correct, we might expect to see those groups that are most vulnerable to the changes in healthcare, including ethnic minorities, the less educated, those in poor health, and the lowest income households, becoming most disillusioned with services. And indeed, an analysis (without any prior controls) of a sample from the GSS shows that there are a few groups where confidence has eroded further and faster than others: women more than men, those living in the south, and those with only high school educations. But the patterns are far from consistent. By the last decade, confidence in medicine was greater among men than women, and it was stronger among those who reported having excellent health. Overall, the differences among social groups are less striking than the similarities. Confidence has eroded in recent decades fairly uniformly among rich and poor, black and white, and among all regions of America.

To examine these patterns more systematically and to see if similar factors predicted confidence in medicine as in other major institutions, ordinary least squares regression analysis models were used with the pooled GSS sample including the year of the survey, the standard social background variables of age, education, race, income, gender, and religiosity, as well as exposure to newspapers and to television, the role of social trust, and the reported satisfaction with the respondent's health. For comparison, a similar model was analyzed using the Confidence in Institutions scale, which summed trust in nine institutions, excluding medicine (Table 3.1). The results of the multivariate analysis show that five factors were

Table 3.1. Models explaining confidence in institutions and in medicine

	Confidence in Institutions				Confidence in Medicine			
	B	Std. Error	Beta	Sig	B	Std. Error	Bet	Sig
(Constant)	197	31.5		.000	7.029	2.520		.005
Year of survey	−.06	.016	−.046	.000	−.002	.001	−.02	.074
Age of respondent (years)	−.05	.007	−.083	.000	−.004	.000	−.11	.000
Sex (male 1/female 0)	.15	.235	.006	.517	.041	.015	.03	.006
Race (White 1/Black 0)	.14	.343	.044	.671	.071	.023	.00	.446
Education (highest year of school completed)	−.12	.045	−.031	.006	.001	.003	.00	.798
Total family income	−.17	.047	−.044	.000	−.005	.003	−.02	.061
Religiosity (how often R attends religious services)	.48	.044	.111	.000	.012	.003	.05	.000
Exposure to newspapers	.69	.103	.071	.000	.012	.007	.02	.080
Exposure to TV (hours/day watching TV)	.12	.055	.024	.020	.005	.004	.01	.141
Social trust	2.35	.251	.097	.000	.086	.016	.06	.000
Satisfaction with condition of own health					.024	.005	.05	.000
R	.1				.16			
Adjusted R²	.03				.024			

Note: Ordinary least squares regression models presenting the results of the unstandardized coefficients (B), the standard errors, the standardized coefficients (Beta), and their significance (Sig) where the confidence in institutions scale and the confidence in medicine are the dependent variables. The institutional confidence scale is composed of the first ten items listed in Table 3.1, excluding medicine. The scale is standardized to 100 points.

Source: NORC U.S. General Social Survey, 1973–2000, sample pooled by decade.

significantly (at the conventional .05 level) and positively related to confidence in medicine, namely the younger generation and men, as well as religiosity, social trust, and reported satisfactory health. Other factors that were significant at the .10 levels include the year of the survey, family income, and exposure to newspapers (which was positively related to trust in medicine). The number of hours of television watched proved insignificant. Many more factors predicted the institutional confidence scale—indeed, all variables proved significant except for sex and race. The strongest associations were with religiosity, suggesting that regular church attendance was linked to greater support for institutions. Social trust was also moderately strongly related to institutional trust. Nevertheless, some qualifications should be stressed. The significance of these coefficients could be attributed to the generous size of the pooled sample. All were fairly weak, and the overall level of variance (R^2) explained by either of these models proved extremely modest.

Comparative Trends in Institutional Confidence

To see whether the trends in the United States are distinctive or whether there has been a fall in institutional confidence across many countries, we turn to comparative evidence. Previous studies have debated whether or not there has been a significant or long-term erosion of public confidence in modern institutions across different postindustrial societies.[13] Some assert that the figures show a mixed pattern, with no clear trends for any given set of institutions, nations, or periods of time. In some instances, the confidence figures fall, but in others they rise, and in still others they are more or less constant. After examining public confidence in 10 sets of public and private institutions in 14 Western European nations between 1981 and 1990, Listhaug and Wiberg concluded: "The data from the two European Values Surveys do not demonstrate that there has been a widespread decline in the public's confidence in institutions during the 1980s."[14] Although they observed a decline of confidence in "order" institutions, they noted that "confidence in other political institutions is either stable, as in the case of the civil service and parliament, or, as with the education system, has become stronger." Listhaug and Wiberg based their conclusions on data up to 1990. More recent evidence from a wider range of nations suggests that the world may have changed since then. Klingemann demonstrates how support for parliaments suffered a marked erosion during the 1990s, while Inglehart documented a decline in confidence in hierarchical and traditional institutions including the military and the church.[15]

Most studies of confidence in institutions have been confined to Western Europe or North America, but we can compare public opinion in a wider range of postindustrial democracies included in both waves of the World Values Survey (WVS) conducted in the early 1980s (1981–1984) and the early 1990s (1990–1993). These include almost 47,000 respondents in 17 established democracies. This group of nations comprises most of the established democracies in the world, and it is broadly representative because it includes both major economic powers like the United States, West Germany, and Japan as well as smaller social-democratic welfare states such as Belgium and Norway. These nations also possess a wide array of political systems and institutional structures, such as presidential versus parliamentary executives, federal versus unitary states, and consensus versus majoritarian systems, which is important if we are to be able to generalize about systematic variations in institutional confidence. The WVS used a four-point response scale for the following question: "Please look at this card and tell me, for each item, how much confidence you have in them. Is it a great deal (4), quite a lot (3), not very much (2) or none at all (1)?" The survey compared public support for 10 institutions, which can be classified as public-sector institutions, understood as those most closely associated with the core functions of the state (including parliament, the civil service, the legal system, the police, and the army), and other institutions in the private and nonprofit sectors (the education system, the church, major companies, trade unions, and the press).[16] Two scales were developed from this data, one for public and one for private institutions.[17]

Cross-national comparison on the basis of these scales confirms a striking and important pattern. During the 1980s, confidence in public institutions declined consistently, if in varying degrees, in all but one society (Iceland). In contrast, the pattern of confidence in private institutions proved more mixed. It fell significantly in Finland, the United States, and Britain, but increased significantly in Spain, Italy, Denmark, West Germany, and France. Based on this evidence, we conclude that there are important cross-national variations in confidence in particular public and private institutions, as we would expect, in terms of both the level of confidence and the direction of trends over time. Although this shows clearly that there is no general loss of support for all social institutions in the countries under comparison, the evidence does indicate declining confidence in public institutions in virtually all nations during the 1980s. The political and governmental problems that have been so widely discussed in the United States are not sui generis but are evident to a greater or lesser extent elsewhere.

Attitudes Toward Doctors

Although confidence in medicine has eroded over recent decades in the United States, reflecting broader patterns of declining trust that are found in many institutions in many societies, has this influenced public opinion toward doctors? Here we lack systematic time series data from either the WVS or from the General Social Survey (GSS), but the latter monitored attitudes using a wide range of indicators in 1998. The results in Table 3.2 show that attitudes vary widely depending upon the particular statement, but overall the results provide relatively positive news for the profession. There was widespread agreement with the statement "I trust my doctor's judgment about my medical care" (81 percent agreed or agreed strongly, and with the statement "I trust my doctor to put my medical needs above all other considerations when treating my medical problems.") By contrast, most of the negative statements about doctors received little support, although the public was more evenly divided on a few items, such as how well doctors explained medical problems to patients, their respect for patients, and their use of surgery.

Table 3.2. Attitudes toward doctors (1998)

	% Agree or Agree Strongly
My doctor is willing to refer me to a specialist when needed.	86
I trust my doctor's judgments about my medical care.	81
I trust my doctor to put my medical needs above all other considerations when treating my medical problems.	74
My doctor would tell me if a mistake was made.	62
My doctor is a real expert in taking care of my problem.	61
Doctors do their best to prevent patients' worrying.	52
Doctors aren't as thorough as they should be.	51
Doctors always treat their patients with respect.	51
Doctors never recommend surgery (an operation) unless there is no other way to solve the problem.	44
Doctors cause people to worry a lot because they don't explain medical problems to patients.	41
Sometimes doctors take unnecessary risks in treating their patients.	35
Doctors are very careful to check everything when examining their patients.	34
I worry that I will be denied the treatment or services I need.	24
I worry that my doctor will put cost considerations above the care I need.	24
Doctors avoid unnecessary patient expenses.	22
I worry that my doctor is being prevented from telling me the full range of options for my treatment.	22
My doctor does not do everything for me.	20
I hardly ever see the same doctor when I go for medical care.	19
The medical problems I've had in the past are ignored when I seek care for a new medical problem.	18
I doubt that my doctor really cares about me as a person.	16

Note: Q.: "As you read each of the following statements, please think about the medical care you are now receiving. If you have not received any medical care recently, circle the answer based on what you would expect if you had to seek care today. Even if you are not entirely certain about your answers, we want to remind you that your best guess is important for each statement. Do you agree strongly, agree, are you uncertain, or do you disagree or disagree strongly?"

Source: NORC U.S. General Social Survey, 1998. Adapted and updated from Pippa Norris, presentation at The Public's Health: A Matter of Trust Symposium, 2002, Harvard University School of Public Health.

Moreover, when asked in a September 2002 survey by Gallup about trust in various information sources about health and medicine, despite the multiplicity of information sources that are now available in print, on the airwaves, and online, doctors remained by far the most trusted source (Table 3.3). Nurses and books were the next most trusted sources, followed by the Internet. And although newspapers, magazines, and television are inundated with ads for drug companies,

Table 3.3. Trusted information sources about health

	Doctors	Nurses	Book	Internet	Magazine	N
A great deal	61	38	36	20	13	1
Moderate amount	32	45	46	42	49	5
Not much	5	10	42	14	23	2
None at all	2	6	5	17	12	1
Don't know	—	1	1	7	3	1

Note: Q.: "How much trust and confidence would you have in information about health and medicine that you could get from each of the following sources?"

Source: Gallup Organization, September 8, 2002, National adult telephone survey N. 1004. Adapted and updated from Pippa Norris, presentation at The Public's Health: A Matter of Trust Symposium, 2002, Harvard University School of Public Health.

mass media were regarded as the least trustworthy sources of information on these subjects.

Conclusions

The results of this study suggest certain important clues about the nature and consequences of declining trust in healthcare, and confirm that confidence in medicine has indeed eroded in the United States during the last three decades, as many claim. Yet trends must be kept in balance: many indicators suggest that, even if faith in medicine has eroded, overall levels of trust in physicians remains relatively high.

Moreover, far from being a problem that is specific to healthcare, this pattern is shown to reflect trends in many other comparable institutions in the private, nonprofit, and public sectors, including education, unions, organized religion, Congress and the Executive branch, the military, major companies, and the mass media. Social trust is associated with institutional confidence, but only weakly. The analysis suggests that a long-term process of value change has altered traditional attitudes toward medicine that lie at the heart of the patient-physician relationship in the United States, as well in other postindustrial societies. The most convincing explanation for this phenomenon focuses on long-term changes in the culture, notably rising cognitive levels and less deference toward authority, rather than on shortcomings evident in the delivery of healthcare per se or a puzzling failure of performance afflicting all major institutions in American society. The study found that the erosion of faith in medicine is not restricted to specific social sectors, such as African Americans, the poor, or those with health problems, but instead occurs fairly uniformly throughout all major groups.

Nor does the frequently discussed tendency of the mass media to report scandal, corruption, and disaster provide an adequate explanation. Although the amount of time people spend watching television entertainment is associated with some indicators of political apathy and disaffection, viewing television news and reading newspapers is also associated with civic mobilization and support for political institutions. Consistent with other research, the evidence in this study shows that regular newspaper readers expressed greater than average confidence in institutions, not less. Regular newspaper reading and television watching were not significantly related to lower levels of trust in medicine. Thus, we have to look elsewhere for plausible explanations.

It is important that the evidence demonstrates a loss of confidence in many public and private institutions, not just medicine, suggesting that the cause lies beyond a simple change in healthcare performance. This makes the search for causes both easier and more difficult. It suggests that the problem is a general cultural shift that affects all or many aspects of modern life. Therefore, the cultural theories of societal modernization provide a more satisfactory explanation of this phenomenon, rather than any specific change in the organization of medicine associated with the introduction of managed care.

Interpreting the implications of these developments, especially from the perspective of the general public, is not straightforward. Medical professionals often regard the rise of more skeptical patients as detrimental to healthcare. Yet, alternative interpretations suggest that, from a societal perspective, this development should not necessarily be regarded as wholly negative. Further research is required to explore the consequences of these developments, but these trends may have led to less deference toward the authority of medical professionals and less willingness to follow medical advice blindly. Patients now may have the cognitive skills necessary to understand more technical medical matters; they may be more motivated to learn about a range of traditional and alternative health options from diverse information sources; and they may also be more demanding of healthcare now. Social changes may have thereby undermined more paternalistic models of medicine. Patients will act differently if they are skeptical of medicine, and healthcare professionals must respond to these changes. Some will regard this as a threat, and others as an opportunity. How the profession responds is one of the challenges facing medicine in the twenty-first century.

Notes

1. See, for example, Francis Fukuyama, *Trust: The Social Virtues and the Creation of Prosperity* (New York: The Free Press, 1995); Russell Hardin, *Trust and Trustworthiness* (New York: Russell Sage, 2002); and Adam Seligman, *The Problem of Trust* (Princeton, N.J.: Princeton University Press, 2000).

2. B. A. Pescosolido, S. A. Tuch, and J. K. Martin, "The Profession of Medicine and the Public: Examining American's Changing Confidence in Physician Authority from the Beginning of the 'Healthcare Crisis' to the Era of Healthcare Reform," *Journal of Health and Social Behavior* 42 (2001): 1–16; M. Schlesinger, "A Loss of Faith: The Sources of Reduced Political Legitimacy for the American Medical Profession," *Milbank Quarterly* 80 (2002): 185–195; D. Mechanic, "Changing Medical Organization and the Erosion of Trust," *Milbank Quarterly* 74 (1996): 171–190; D. Mechanic, "The Functions and Limitations of Trust in the Provision of Medical Care," *Journal of Health Politics, Policy, and*

Law 23 (1998): 661–686; and C. C. Clark, "Trust in Medicine," *Journal of Medicine and Philosophy* 27 (2002): 11–29.

3. P. Illingworth, "Trust: The Scarcest of Medical Resources," *Journal of Medicine and Philosophy* 27 (2002): 31–46.

4. E. J. Emanuel and N. N. Dubler, "Preserving the Physician-Patient Relationship in the Era of Managed Care," *Journal of the American Medical Association* 273 (1995): 323–329.

5. D. Mechanic, "Changing Medical Organization"; D. Mechanic, "The Functions and Limitations"; D. Mechanic and M. Schlesinger, "The Impact of Managed Care on Patients' Trust in Medical Care and Their Physicians," *Journal of the American Medical Association* 275 (1996): 1693–1697.

6. See Robert D. Putnam, *Making Democracy Work* (Princeton, N.J.: Princeton University Press, 1994); Robert D. Putnam, "Bowling Alone: America's Declining Social Capital," *Journal of Democracy* 6 (1995): 65–78; Robert D. Putnam, "Tuning In, Tuning Out: The Strange Disappearance of Social Capital in America," *P.S.: Political Science and Politics* 28 (1995): 664–683; Robert D. Putnam, *Bowling Alone* (New York: Simon & Schuster, 2000). See also V. A. Braithwaite and Margaret Levi, eds., *Trust and Governance* (New York: Russell Sage, 1998); and Mark Warren, ed., *Democracy and Trust* (New York: Cambridge University Press, 1999).

7. For a short summary of current knowledge about social capital and its application to health policy, see S. E. Shortt, "Making Sense of Social Capital, Health and Policy," *Health Policy* 70 (2004): 11–22.

8. For an interdisciplinary analysis of the role trust plays in health system relationships, see L. Gilson, "Trust and the Development of Health Care as a Social Institution," *Social Science and Medicine* 56 (2003): 1453–1468.

9. For an example of a study depicting this relationship, see M. M. Ahern and M. S. Hendryx, "Social Capital and Trust in Providers," *Social Science and Medicine* 57 (2003): 1195–1203.

10. See Ronald Inglehart, *Culture Shift in Advanced Industrial Society* (Princeton, N.J.: Princeton University Press, 1990); Ronald Inglehart and Christian Welzel, *Modernization and Postmodernization: Cultural, Economic and Political Change in 43 Societies* (Princeton, N.J.: Princeton University Press, 1997); Ronald Inglehart, *The Silent Revolution: Changing Values and Political Styles among Western Publics* (Princeton, N.J.: Princeton University Press, 1977); Ronald Inglehart, "The Erosion of Institutional Authority and Post-Materialist Values," in *Why Americans Mistrust Government,* ed. Joseph S. Nye, Philip D. Zelikow, and David C. King (Cambridge, Mass.: Harvard University Press, 1997); Ronald Inglehart, "Postmodernization Erodes Support for Authority but Increases Support for Democracy," in *Critical Citizens: Global Support for Democratic Governance,* ed. Pippa Norris (New York: Oxford University Press, 1999); and Ronald Inglehart and Pippa Norris, *Rising Tide: Gender Equality and Cultural Change around the World* (New York: Cambridge University Press, 2003).

11. D. H. Thom, K. M. Ribisl, A. L. Stewart, and D. A. Luke, "Further Validation and Reliability Testing of the Trust in Physician Scale," *Medical Care* 37 (1999): 510–517. For discussion of other attempts, see D. H. Thom, M. A. Hall, and L. G. Pawlson, "Measuring Patients' Trust in Physicians When Assessing Quality of Care," *Health Affairs* 23 (2004): 124–132; and A. Rose, N. Petyers, J. A. Shea et al., "Development and Testing of the Health Care System Distrust Scale," *Journal of General Internal Medicine* 19 (2004): 57–63.

12. Seymour M. Lipset and William C. Schneider, *The Confidence Gap: Business, La-*

·   *bor, and Government in the Public Mind,* rev. ed. (Baltimore: Johns Hopkins University
Press, 1987).

    13. See Ola Listhaug and Matti Wiberg, "Confidence in Political and Private Institutions," in *Citizens and the State,* ed. Hans-Dieter Klingemann and Dieter Fuchs (Oxford: Oxford University Press, 1995); Joseph Nye, Philip D. Zelikow, and David C. King, eds., *Why People Don't Trust Government* (Cambridge: Harvard University Press, 1997).

    14. Listhaug and Wiberg, "Confidence in Political and Private Institutions."

    15. See Klingemann and Fuchs, *Citizens;* Inglehart, "Postmodernization"; and Norris, ed., *Critical Citizens.*

    16. As previous studies have suggested, it should be noted that the precise dividing line between state and nonstate institutions is not clear-cut. The education system is often largely but not exclusively within the public sector, for example. In the same way, established churches can be seen as part of the state. This study nevertheless distinguishes between those institutions that can be regarded as most closely associated with the functions of the state and those in the nonprofit and public sectors.

    17. The measures of confidence in the 10 institutions were summed to form two consistent 20-point scales measuring confidence in public institutions and confidence in private institutions. These scales proved suitable for analysis because the separate items were highly intercorrelated, producing scales with a normal and nonskewed distribution with high reliability (Cronbach's Alpha = .77 for the confidence in public institutions scale and .66 for the confidence in private institutions scale).

II

Quality and Safety:
The Basics of Trust

4

Building Quality in the
Healthcare Environment

DONALD M. BERWICK

Quality and trust are first cousins. If a mechanic fixes your car to your satisfaction, if a teacher helps you learn Spanish, or if a doctor cures your illness, you trust them. If they fail to help you—if they do not deliver on their promises, whether explicit or implicit—you trust them less. In short, *results build trust.* The fastest way to improve the trust level in healthcare may be to improve the performance of the healthcare system.

But performance improvement, to put it mildly, is no small task. If it were easy, we would not suffer from the serious quality problems that continue to plague medicine in the United States. Peculiarities of the healthcare system make change exceptionally challenging, cumbersome, and time-consuming. Interestingly, a high level of trust could play a key role in the process of change itself.[1]

That the healthcare system has serious quality issues will come as no news to researchers working in the field. Study after study during the past 40 years has documented the system's gaps and failings. In recent years, some of the leading institutions in healthcare have stamped their imprimaturs on these findings. In 1998, the National Roundtable on Healthcare Quality, sponsored by the Institute of Medicine (IOM), weighed in with a lead article in the *Journal of the American Medical Association.*

> Serious and widespread quality problems exist throughout American medicine. These problems . . . occur in small and large communities alike, in all parts of the country, and with approximately equal frequency in managed care and fee-for-service systems of care. Very large numbers of Americans are harmed as a result.[2]

About the same time, both the National Cancer Policy Board and the President's Advisory Commission on Consumer Protection and Quality in the Healthcare Industry issued unsettling findings about the quality of care in the United States.[3] In 2001, the IOM issued its massive report *Crossing the Quality Chasm: A New Health System for the Twenty-First Century.* Similar studies have emerged in many other countries, including Australia, the United Kingdom, and the Scandinavian nations. Together, these comprehensive summary statements provide a kind of certification that the status quo in healthcare is unsatisfactory.

It is beyond the scope of this chapter to examine these quality problems in detail. The IOM Roundtable lumped many of them into three categories: overuse of procedures that do not help people get better; underuse of procedures that can help; and misuse, or errors. In the overuse category, for example, a Colorado study found that 30 percent of children receive excessive antibiotics for ear infections. The RAND Corporation has reported that between 20 percent and 50 percent of many surgical operations are unnecessary. In back pain patients, as many as 50 percent of X-rays are unnecessary. Examples of underuse include the finding that 50 percent of elderly patients fail to receive pneumococcal vaccine, while 50 percent of heart attack victims fail to receive beta blockers. Misuse, or medical error, is a topic dealt with at greater length in chapter 5. It suffices to say that nearly 7 percent of hospital patients each year experience a serious medication error.[4]

Another lens on quality of care—beyond overuse, underuse, and misuse—is clinical results. One example is cystic fibrosis (CF). The Cystic Fibrosis Foundation in Bethesda, Maryland, collects data on every child with the disease who has been treated in 160 cystic fibrosis centers throughout the United States. The foundation examines many outcomes of care and compares the national average with the range among these centers. The variation in outcomes is striking. Nationally, for example, about 26 percent of children with CF are below the tenth percentile for weight. Yet the range among centers is from 7.4 percent to 60 percent. Nationally, the median length of hospital stay for children under 18 is 9.7 days. The range among centers is from 2.5 days to 16.5 days. The national average for FEV1 (forced expiratory volume), a measure of lung function, is 73.5 percent of the predicted normal value. The range among centers is from 70.1 percent to 104.4 percent for children ages 6 to 13, and from 40.0 percent to 85.8 percent for adults ages 18 to 30.

Changing the System

With the growing use of information technologies and measurement in healthcare, results-oriented data sets like these are now out of the bottle; the genie has escaped. And the public is demanding, or will soon demand, change. But how can the healthcare system change? Everyone has an opinion about this emotionally charged sector of our economy and society. It is an entrenched system of institutions, training, and behaviors, with deeply embedded rules and beliefs. Moreover, providing healthcare is a difficult, demanding job for clinicians and healthcare workers of all sorts, from managed care executives to hospital orderlies, who function in a fishbowl characterized by high expectations, deep personal commitment, and low tolerance for error. Changing the way they deliver services has to be done with caution and with great respect for the contexts in which they work.

And yet, change is possible. Other industries, almost as large and as cumbersome as healthcare, have changed substantially during the last couple of decades.

Automobile manufacturers, for instance, reorganized the way they operate in response to the competition from Japan. Healthcare can already point to some successful examples of change. The key is that change must start from the right premises.

When changing performance, the most crucial premise is this: *Quality is a system property.* In its own small way, this is a revolutionary notion, swimming upstream against strong cultural habits. Not long ago, for example, *USA Today* ran a front-page story headlined "Is Your Doctor Bad? You May Never Know." The article was a reasonable plea for greater access to data about medical errors. Underlying it, however, was a strong and erroneous theory about the solution to quality problems in healthcare, namely, find the bad doctors and get rid of them. To be sure, everybody acknowledges the existence of a few problem doctors and a few badly run healthcare institutions. But the variation in outcomes our data show us cannot possibly be accounted for by a few bad apples, nor by a few exceptionally good ones. What determines the level of quality is the design of a system, not a group of individuals within that system.

The notion that quality is a system property may be revolutionary, but it isn't hard to grasp. If you buy a new car—a Ford Windstar, for example—you will find that your car has a certain top speed. You can take it out on the Bonneville Salt Flats and floor the accelerator. If its top speed does not please you, you can get angry at it for not going faster. You can give it incentives. You can put an incident report in its file. None of this, of course, will change its performance: the car will never go faster than it is able, and if you want to go faster, you need a different kind of car. So it is with all the data on quality and results of care. The patient mortality rate of a hospital and all the other outcomes that we care about are properties of a certain system at work. There is a saying among people who study this kind of thing: "Every system is perfectly designed to achieve exactly the results it gets." I call this the First Law of Improvement.[5] If you want a better result, you have to change the system.[6]

How do you change a system? The first key premise is that those seeking change must face reality. It does no good to say we have to change without understanding where you stand now or the difference between where you are now and where you want to be. The second premise is that you must be interested in new designs. If you want to go faster than a Windstar allows, you must find or build a car *designed* to go faster. If cost is a constraint, you must see if there are any cars designed to go faster for the same money, or you must design one from scratch. The third premise is that everyone must be involved in the change. An individual can learn tennis or Spanish alone or with a teacher. But individual healthcare practitioners cannot learn to lower mortality rates, cut costs, or reduce error rates by themselves. They need to work on the problems together. They are a team, whether they know it or not.

The goal of change is to improve results. But trust is required before the process of change can begin. People trying to improve must trust that the future, though unknown, can be better than the known present. If that trust fails, they have no reason to go forward. Patients and patients' families need to be trusted.

Instead of blaming patients for expecting that the healthcare system will in fact help them, we need to enlist their aid in figuring out how it can do so better. We must also trust ourselves, have confidence in our own ability to deal with a difficult environment. People in healthcare, like people everywhere, may find it easier to blame others for their troubles. Healthcare has many promising targets for blame: insurance companies, the government, regulators, lawyers, and the media. But the blame game is nonsense.[7] It is an escape from responsibility. It would be incomparably more productive for providers to move the perceived locus of control to an internal one. Yes, the policy world is tough and will remain so; the environment is hostile and will remain so; the lawyers are doing their jobs the way they are trained. All those realities are not likely to change. But at the end of the day, it is our responsibility to effect change, and we have the power to do so.

There is one last, critically important form of trust—trust in the workforce. The people who provide and arrange for healthcare have to be the people who change it. They must trust themselves to do so and must be trusted to do so.

Beyond Taylorism

When it comes to change in the workplace, we are handicapped by a widespread, often implicit, theory of production—a theory of the workforce. It is often called Taylorism, after Frederick W. Taylor, though in many ways the label is unfair. Taylor's thinking was complex and deep, and his aims were often laudable. The management system that bears his name does not do the man justice. But if we want to understand how to change the workplace, we must understand and question many of the principles of Taylorism.

Frederick Winslow Taylor was born in 1856 to a well-to-do Philadelphia family. Unlike other young men of his background, he dropped out of Harvard and went to work in a metal-products factory as a machinist. In the course of his career, he became a self-taught industrial engineer, and he had a groundbreaking insight about production and production workers. At the time, industrial production was new. Much of the work done in factories was based on an earlier craft model of production, which is to say that skilled employees performed a variety of tasks, often manufacturing parts or products from start to finish. Taylor thought that if the work could be subdivided into highly specialized tasks, it could be performed by less skilled workers.[8] He also timed employees as they performed their tasks and to arrange the workflow to maximize the output of each worker and of the factory as a whole. *Scientific management,* as his system became known, rigorously separated the planning of the work done by engineers such as Taylor from the execution of the work by laborers.[9] Workers on the shop floor performed their tasks as fast as they could and exactly as they were told, no more and no less.

Taylor's system meshed perfectly with two other developments in industrialization. One was the use of interchangeable parts, pioneered in government armories as early as 1820 but adopted only gradually by U.S. industry over the ensuing decades. The other was the moving assembly line, pioneered by Henry

Ford in the beginning of the twentieth century. Thanks to Taylor and other innovators, it was not long before factories such as Ford's were operating on what we were raised to view as modern industrial principles. Workers had bins of wheels and axles and all the other parts that went into a car. Each part was manufactured to specifications. Each worker did one small series of tasks as the line moved along. The result of specialization was that factories turned out masses of standardized goods far, far cheaper than ever before. Costs fell. Quality rose. Suddenly, most Americans could afford a car. It was a momentous achievement.

But there was a price to pay. Each worker became no more than a pair of hands. Taylor was deeply respectful of labor and laborers and indeed viewed his system as enabling workers to attain a higher standard of living than they otherwise could. He wanted them to express their individuality at home, not at work. In the factory, the worker's job was to follow the rules in manuals and enforced by supervisors. If a worker had an idea about how to build a better axle, he should keep it to himself; after all, the new axle might not fit the standard. There would be innovation, of course. But innovation was the responsibility of the engineers and planners, not the laborers. As for quality, that was primarily the responsibility of inspectors. In 1925, one-fourth of the employees at Western Electric labs, which made telephone equipment, were inspectors. The inspection system worked well enough—quality was fairly good, in general—but it was not likely to improve much from one month to the next, because the system was not focused on improvement.[10]

Healthcare came late to the Taylorist party. For most of the last century, the model for healthcare delivery was very much a craft model. Individual doctors would treat the patient using their professional skills, experience, and judgment. In the 1980s, perhaps influenced by the evidence-based medicine movement, providers became interested in developing detailed protocols for care, and so created Taylor-like standards for many procedures. The Harvard anesthesia guidelines, for instance, spelled out a precise series of steps for anesthesiologists to follow: connect the oxygen, don't leave the room, and so on. Much of this helped. Many parts of medicine should be Taylorized, spelled out in protocols and followed to the letter. No parents want an anesthesiologist experimenting with new and untried procedures when their child is in the operating room. "Healthcare," a Baldrige award judge said to me in 1989, "has discovered Frederick Taylor and fallen in love."

But while healthcare was discovering Taylorism, other industries were moving well beyond it. The auto industry is a notable example. Influenced—and threatened—by Japanese competition, the car companies and other large manufacturers began experimenting with a wholly different approach to work and the workplace. The key principles of this new approach are in many ways the exact opposite of what Taylor and his disciples taught. Taylor and Ford expected every customer to take what they produced. ("The customer can have any color Model T he likes, as long as it's black" was Ford's famous dictum.) In the new view, every customer is an individual with individual needs and preferences, and quality consists of meeting those needs and preferences. Taylor and Ford assumed that there was a tradeoff between quality and cost. In the new view, improving quality usually reduces costs. Taylor and Ford assumed that quality could be improved only in chunks, when the engineers designed improvements. In the new view, quality can be improved continually, thanks to incremental changes originating on the shop floor.[11] Underlying this new approach is the fundamental premise that quality and cost are inherent in processes. They are properties of a system. If you want to improve quality and lower cost, you must change the processes that make up the system.

The new view also has a different idea of the employee's role. Taylor espoused only one kind of role for employees: understand what you are supposed to do and do it. The new approach assumes that everyone is likely to have ideas for process improvement, and the more ideas you get, the more likely you are to improve the processes. Since the best foundation for change is trying something, measuring the result, and learning from the measurement, the employee practices what might be called pragmatic or real-time science aimed at making the work continually more productive. The "hands" that staffed Taylor's factory also have minds, and the intrinsic motivation to improve seems to be abundant in the human mind.[12] Nearly everyone comes to work wanting to do a good job and to feel proud of what they do. Most would probably like to learn a little something as well. And so the energy behind the scientific pursuit of change, behind continuous improvement, is latent in the employees. When leaders and managers tap that energy by providing people the opportunity to improve work, they are tapping into a powerful force.

A Model for Improvement

Of course, understanding that the workforce needs to be engaged in the process of change is only the first step. It does not tell you how to go about it. For that you need what might be called a model for improvement. Some years ago, Thomas W. Nolan and his colleagues laid out one of the best.[13] The model asks three questions: What are we trying to accomplish? How will we know that a change is an improvement? What changes can we make that will result in an improvement? Once a team has answers to these questions, it can test changes to see what works and what fails to work.

What Are We Trying to Accomplish?

All improvement requires a goal, an aim. This precept is not so different from the need to face reality, as described earlier. Nobody learns Spanish until he (a) acknowledges that he does not already know Spanish and (b) decides that he wants to learn it. In a Taylorist workplace, the workforce by definition has no aim other than getting the job done and collecting a paycheck. In a post-Taylorist workplace, the workforce has to develop the skill of *identifying and agreeing on what they are going to make better.*

This is no small matter. An organization's leaders must acknowledge and publicly recognize the difference between where an organization is and where it wants to be. That gap must be measured. What is more, it must be measured and communicated publicly; if it is done in secret, people will be inclined to forget about it or rationalize it away. One way to identify and measure a gap, or an aim, is simply to listen to people. Talk to patients. Talk to their families. Talk to employees. Study the effect of the organization's work on the people it is trying to help. That, incidentally, involves a high level of trust. There is no point in asking somebody how we are doing, if you do not trust the validity of their answer. A second technique is simply to scrutinize the numbers. A cystic fibrosis center, for instance, could compare the percentage of its children under the tenth percentile for weight with the distribution of those numbers among all CF centers. An aim most often comes from numbers, not from philosophy. And it comes from the specific belief—trust, again—that we, as a team, can close that gap.

Of course, whenever anyone proposes an improvement in a complex system, competing ideas emerge about what else should be improved. The report *Crossing the Quality Chasm* listed six categories for improvement: safety, effectiveness, patient-centeredness, timeliness, efficiency, and equity. Any one hospital might want to improve tuberculosis care or AIDS care or waiting times, or indeed pursue a host of other objectives. So, part of developing the skills for pursuing an aim is developing the ability to confront and resolve conflicts about what will be done first. That, too, involves trust.

How Will We Know That a Change Is an Improvement?

All improvement is change, but not all change is improvement. You know you are at least on the right track when the numbers move in the right direction. Even there, however, identifying a true improvement can require sophisticated interpretation of variation and covariation. Is 10 percent really better than 8 percent, for example, or is that empirical difference simply within the range of random fluctuation? Have we adequately controlled for extraneous variables so that—in comparing death rates, say—we are actually comparing apples to apples? Are we examining changes in cost at the same time that we are examining changes in outcomes? Also, measurements usually must be conducted over time to be helpful in assessing improvement. What matters is not simply a single number—an average or cross section; it is a trend over time, allowing us to study the direction in which performance is heading. As important as the numbers, of course, are the words, the narratives. What is happening at ground level because of the change? Do the people affected by the change believe that it is really an improvement?

What Changes Can We Make That Will Result in Improvement?

The third part of the model is actually to find the right change. Cincinnati Children's Hospital Medical Center (CCHMC) began a project to improve its cystic fibrosis care because its CF kids were only in the thirtieth percentile nationally in nutritional status. The staff's job was to find the best centers and crawl all over them to find out what they were doing differently. Supported by the Robert Wood Johnson's *Project Perfection: Raising the Bar for Health Care Performance,* Cincinnati Children's implemented a system where adolescent patients and their families fully participate in the design and implementation of their treatment regimen. The result was a dramatic increase patient cooperation, treatment compliance, and health outcomes. Encouraged by its effort to improve the quality of treatment for cystic fibrosis, CCHMC has taken steps to render care for other diseases (*e.g.,* diabetes mellitus, juvenile rheumatoid arthritis, bronchitis) more family-centered and evidence-based.[14]

There is no way around this kind of research. Third parties, no matter how eminent, cannot do this effectively or efficiently. It has to be done by the people who are trying to improve, and it is often best done in groups. A team from Cincinnati has to go to Michigan or wherever the best centers are located, spend several days at each one, and walk through their process. Nor can this information be gathered in secret. The exchange of information has to be open, and it has to be two-way, so that the people being examined can learn from the examiners as well. The fundamental skill is what I call authentic curiosity. The team has to ask how do you really do this? How do you do so much better than we do? They have to mean it, and they have to want to hear the answer. Trust is central to this entire endeavor. If the questions are asked with distrust, with distance, they will not be authentic. And the answers will not be heard when they are offered.

The searchers, moreover, must cast a wide net. Not all of the answers will lie in other healthcare organizations. Right now, for instance, we could eliminate many of the waits and delays in hospitals and clinics. The resources are available. But the current models of scheduling and flow management in healthcare do not work; they have delays embedded in them. The best models for continuous flow lie in other industries, not in healthcare. Healthcare people must venture beyond the boundaries of their professions to discover them.

Run a Test of Change

When my daughter was learning to ride a bike, thinking about the task was not enough. She also had to practice until she learned all the muscle movements and techniques and made them her own. Improving healthcare is no different. Plan/do/study/act (PDSA) means running real-world tests of change and learning from what happens. People in an organization need to develop the skills to run many tests, assess the results, and make changes accordingly.

A handful of basic rules govern effective use of the PDSA cycle. The tests are best conducted in teams, so that learning takes place among a whole group. They must be adapted to local conditions, which will not be the same in Maine as they are in Minnesota. A key rule is that small and frequent tests are better than big and slow ones. In formal science, tests are often large scale and take a lot of time. That is often as it should be. In real-time science, on the ground, the best tests are small, quick, and frequent. We have a saying in the Institute for Healthcare Improvement: What test will you run next Tuesday? That is a reminder that prompt improvements require actually making changes, right now, in a matter of days, rather than over a period of months or years. Real change requires performing dozens, hundreds, of tests, over and over.

Another key rule is that you must be open and honest about "failed" tests, which are often the most valuable. After all, what is a failed test? The tester learns that something did not work. All that means is that the next test will be different and perhaps will lead the investigators closer to the desired result. It is natural for human beings to want to forget about experiments that do not work. But any scientist knows that the learning from failures is just as important as the learning from successes. You rule out attractive but unproductive hypotheses. You identify unexpected correlations and consequences. You get smarter.

Facing Reality (Once More)

Making improvement work, in the end, requires a mindset different from the status quo. The Japanese have two words that describe the old mindset and the new, and they are worth learning. *Taseki* means "your burden." In this context, it means claiming that the problem is anybody else's but mine. Imagine that you and your colleagues are looking at some performance numbers, perhaps numbers that show a serious gap between where you are and where you would like to be. The initial reaction is usually "The data are wrong." And the second reaction is usually "The data are right, but it's not a problem." It is not much of a jump to the third reaction, which is "The data are right, and it's a problem—but it's not *my* problem!" *Taseki* is a way of saying "The dog ate my homework." It isn't my fault. It isn't my responsibility.

The term *jiseki* means the opposite, "my responsibility." It means I've got it. I will do it. I accept responsibility. As mentioned earlier, it involves not blaming cost constraints, the environment, the regulators, or anybody else for the current state of affairs, and it means accepting the responsibility for making change. *Jiseki* is a tough mindset. Once you accept responsibility for gaps, for example, you feel guilty right away. You have to have faith—trust—in yourself that you are not bad, you are good, and that you can get better. You will experience a fear of failure, another obstacle that you must have the faith to overcome. Psychologically, *taseki* is much easier!

Jiseki also exposes you to attacks, both internally and externally. If you admit the problem and accept responsibility for it, the question Why haven't you solved it already? immediately arises. Sometimes there are explanations. For example, why hasn't the American Hospital Association come forward and embraced the six aims of the IOM report as its strategic agenda? Why hasn't it set a national improvement plan for hospital care?[15] To do so, of course, could weaken the organization's political leverage in Washington. It is hard to say simultaneously that we take responsibility for our failings, and by the way, we need a lot more money. Inside an organization, the task is equally hard. Plenty of people will tell you that they are doing their best, that they are working as hard as they can, and that you cannot expect them to do any more. They are right. What they may not realize at first is that, according to the First Law of Improvement, you do not want them to do more, you want them to do things differently.

Ultimately, change requires leadership. Healthcare is a stressed industry, and productivity is on everybody's minds. Yet the leader must say, "Improvement is a requirement, not an option, and all improvement is change." That involves high levels of trust in both directions, from leader to led and back again. *Taseki* requires no trust, just an ability to offload your problems onto someone else. *Jiseki* requires high trust and hard work.[16] But it is the only road to a better future.

Acknowledgment

An earlier version of these ideas appeared as "Improvement, Trust, and the Health-care Workforce," *Quality and Safety in Health Care* 12, suppl 1 (2003): I2–I6.

Notes

1. Donald Berwick, "The Importance and Paucity of Trust in Today's Health Care System," *Trustee* 58, no. 4 (2005): 32–34.

2. M. R. Chassin, R. W. Galvin, and the National Roundtable on Healthcare Quality, "The Urgent Need to Improve Healthcare Quality," *Journal of the American Medical Association* 280 (1998): 1000–1005.

3. M. Hewitt and J. V. Simone, eds., *Ensuring Quality Cancer Care* (Washington, D.C.: National Academy Press, 1999); and The Advisory Commission on Consumer Protection and Quality in the Healthcare Industry, *Quality First: Better Healthcare for All Americans: Final Report to the President of the United States* (Washington, D.C.: U.S. Government Printing Office, 1998).

4. Institute of Medicine, Committee on Quality of Health Care in America, *To Err Is Human: Building a Safer Health System,* ed. Linda T. Kohn, Janet M. Corrigan, and Molla S. Donaldson, (Washington, D.C.: National Academies Press, 2000).

5. Donald M. Berwick, "A Primer on Leading the Improvement of Systems," *British Medical Journal* 312 (1996): 619–622.

6. For a discussion of both the need for systemic overhaul in healthcare and the difficulties of achieving that aim, see Donald Berwick, Andrea Kabenell, and Thomas Nolan, "No Toyota Yet, But a Start: A Cadre of Providers Seeks to Transform an Inefficient Industry—Before It's Too Late," *Modern Healthcare* 35 (January 31, 2005): 18–19.

7. The desire to escape the adversarial system of justice has prompted several attempts to reform medical malpractice. See K. Ignagni, "Moving Beyond the Blame Game," *Frontiers of Health Service Management* 20, no.1 (2003): 3–14, esp. 12.

8. Frederick W. Taylor summarized his proposals for efficient production systems in *The Principles of Scientific Management* (New York: Harper, 1911).

9. For a discussion of Taylor's differentiation between the "planning of work" and the "execution of work," see Robert Kanigel, *The One Best Way: Frederick Winslow Taylor and the Enigma of Efficiency* (New York: Viking, 1997).

10. During the middle decades of the twentieth century, efficiency experts struggled to find a compromise between the goals of efficiency and innovation. For a general discussion

of this tension in industrial planning, see Stephen P. Waring, *Taylorism Transformed: Scientific Management Theory Since 1945* (Chapel Hill: University of North Carolina Press, 1991).

11. It is unclear that Taylor shared the same premise as Henry Ford. Whereas Ford measured production changes by their immediate costs and benefits, Taylor espoused a more organic model that stressed the importance of constant study and refinement. See Frederick W. Taylor, *Shop Management* (New York: McGraw-Hill, 1911), esp. Introduction.

12. Among historians of manufacturing, there remains debate over the fundamental effects of Taylorized systems, with one camp noting its power to dehumanize workers and devalue their contributions toward innovation. The opposing historiographic school argues that rationalized factory systems fostered the generation of specialized expertise that encouraged employee participation in redesigning production systems. For an elaboration of this debate, see Daniel Nelson, *Frederick W. Taylor and the Rise of Scientific Management* (Madison: University of Wisconsin Press, 1981).

13. Gerald J. Langley, Kevin M. Nolan, Clifford M. Norman, Lloyd P. Provost, and Thomas W. Nolan, *The Improvement Guide: A Practical Approach to Enhancing Organizational Performance* (San Francisco: Jossey Bass, 1996).

14. Cincinnati Children's Hospital Medical Center, "Center for Health Care Quality Established to Improve Care for People Around the World," *2006 Pediatric Health News Releases*, Mar 29, 2006. Available: http://www.cincinnatichildrens.org/about/news/release/2006/3-health-care-quality.htm (Accessed April 18, 2006); Institute for Healthcare Improvement, "Pursuing Perfection: Report from Cincinnati Children's on Improving Family-Centered Care for Cystic Fibrosis Patients," n.d., available: http://www.ihi.org/IHI/Topics/ChronicConditions/AllConditions/ImprovementStories/PursuingPerfectionReport fromCincinnatiChildrensImprovingFamilyCenteredCare.htm (accessed April 12, 2006); and, James Anderson & Uma Kotagal, "Quality in an Academic Setting," *Modern Healthcare* 35 (February 2005): 36–37.

15. Some hospitals and American Hospital Association representatives fear that adopting radically new plans for improving quality might suggest that hospitals were generally unsafe beforehand. See Lisa Greene, "Ambitious Effort Aims to Save 100,000," *St. Petersburg Times* (Florida), April 18, 2005, 1B. In 2005, the AHA launched a center for healthcare quality, but did not specify any concrete plans for meeting the Institute of Medicine's recommendations. See Melanie Evans, "Two Better than One?" *Modern Healthcare* 35 (May 2005): 8–9. One explanation for the AHA's inaction is the lack of consensus as to *how exactly* should implement the IOM's recommendations. See Jeff Tieman, "Who Will Take Charge on Quality," *Modern Healthcare* 34 (January 2004): 30. The American Hospital Association encourages quality, in part, through its annual McKesson Quest for Quality Prize. Yet, because the prize recipients have taken diverse paths toward quality improvement, the AHA may be reluctant to commit to a *national* improvement plan for hospital care. See "Four Hosptials Honored for Commitment to Quality," *American Hospital Association Press Release,* July 27, 2005, available: http://www.aha.org/aha/press_room-info/archive.jsp.

16. Donald M. Berwick, "Improvement, Trust, and the Healthcare Workforce," *Quality and Safety in Health Care* 2003, 12(6): 448–452.

5

Medical Errors and Patient Safety

LUCIAN L. LEAPE

As Donald J. Berwick argues in chapter 4, poor results in healthcare undermine trust. But another trust buster is how providers respond to poor results. What do physicians and healthcare organizations do when faced with medical errors and other adverse events? How are these events communicated to patients? How are problem clinicians dealt with? I believe the best way to build trust in a healthcare setting is to create a culture of safety—a culture in which professionals feel comfortable confronting issues of this sort and addressing them openly and effectively. This chapter examines the principles and practices that provide the foundation for such a culture.

Safety issues appeared on the radar screen of most health professionals rather abruptly, in late 1999. That was when the Institute of Medicine (IOM) issued its groundbreaking report on medical errors, "To Err is Human." Though the report received much publicity, many of the key data were not new. For example, the IOM reported that 44,000 to 98,000 people die each year as a result of medical accidents. The higher figure came from the Medical Practice Study conducted by me and my colleagues in New York state and published in 1991, almost a decade earlier. In that study, we looked at 30,000 medical records of patients hospitalized in acute care hospitals. The goal was to discover if they had experienced an adverse event, which we defined as a disabling injury caused by treatment. When we found such an event, we asked whether it was caused by an error or by negligence, meaning the failure to meet the existing standard of care.

The results are summarized in Table 5.1. More than a thousand patients, or nearly 4 percent of the total, had experienced an adverse event. More than 150, or 0.5 percent, died as a result. But the interesting thing to me was that the majority of adverse events, 69 percent, were caused by errors and were therefore potentially preventable. That encouraged us to think about what we could do about errors.

To put these figures in context, consider some data gathered by the French physician Rene Amalberti, who has been studying what he calls ultrasafe industries (Figure 5.1). Amalberti classifies three different types of enterprises: the

Table 5.1. Medical practice study

Records reviewed	30,000	
Adverse events	1,133	(3.7%)
Deaths	157	(0.5%)
Preventable AE	788	(69.0%)
AE 2° negligence	280	(1.0%)

Source: Leape et al. Incidence of adverse events and negligence in hospitalized patients: results of the Harvard Medical Practice Study I, 1991. Adapted and updated from Lucian L. Leape, MD, presentation at The Public's Health: A Matter of Trust Symposium, 2002, Harvard University School of Public Health.

ultrasafe, which includes aviation, nuclear power, and so on; regulated, which includes driving; and hazardous. The *x*-axis—a logarithmic scale—shows the number of encounters for each fatality. The *y*-axis, also logarithmic, is the total number of fatalities per year. For example, the graph shows that on average, about 300 people die each year in scheduled-airline accidents. The mortality risk for an individual is roughly one in three million. If we use the Medical Practice Study figures, we estimate that about 98,000 people die annually because of preventable medical accidents. The risk is an estimated one in 300.

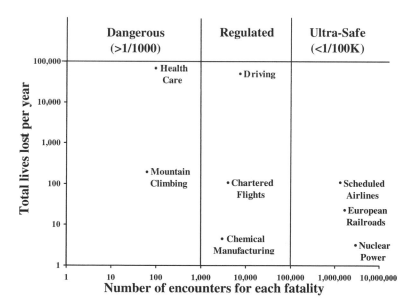

Figure 5.1. How hazardous is health care?

Source: Adapted and updated from Lucian L. Leape, M.D., presentation at The Public's Health: A Matter of Trust Symposium, 2002, Harvard University School of Public Health. Graphics derived from data in R. Amalberti, "The Paradoxes of Almost Totally Safe Transportation Systems," *Safety Science* 36, no. 1 (2000): 1–18.

These numbers describe a major problem. Even if you quibble about their accuracy—if you want to cut them in half, say—they are still horrendous and impossible to ignore. Moreover, the New York Medical Practice Study has been replicated elsewhere. A study in Colorado and Utah produced slightly lower figures. Studies in Australia, the United Kingdom, Denmark, and New Zealand came up with significantly higher numbers, perhaps because these countries maintain better records (and their doctors are less afraid of malpractice suits).

Why are things so bad? One reason is surely that healthcare is the most complicated industry in the world, more complex than making automobiles or designing nuclear reactors or flying airplanes. There are a phenomenally high number of opportunities for things to go wrong. For example, the number of prescriptions written each year was 2.4 billion a couple of years ago, and it has since gone up. A study of prescribing in doctors' offices shows that the prescription error rate is about 10 percent. So there are roughly 240 million errors each year.[1] Most such errors are trivial, such as forgetting to indicate the strength of a drug; usually the pharmacist catches them. But if only 10 percent of those errors are serious enough to cause some kind of adverse event, that leaves 24 million serious errors. We know from hospital studies of serious errors that about one in five such errors actually results in an injury. If that ratio holds, then these prescription errors would lead to 4.8 million adverse events. How many of these would be fatal we simply do not know, but it would not be a trivial number. Very small error rates in very large numbers produce a sizable number of injuries and deaths.

Confronted by such numbers, people react in a variety of ways. Typically, they look for alternative explanations and resolutions of the problem. In particular, they fall back on what might be called the Three Myths of Medical Errors. The first myth is that the numbers are wrong; the problem can't possibly be that bad. This belief, unfortunately, cannot stand up against the evidence. Enough studies have been conducted to show that the estimates above are probably low, not high. The second myth is that, even if there is a problem, nobody knows what to do about it. That is false as well. Several years ago, for instance, the American Hospital Association distributed a list of 13 best practices for medication safety, yet there probably is not a single hospital in the country that has implemented all 13. The third myth is that there aren't enough resources to implement safety measures. What is wrong with this idea, of course, is that some hospitals have much better safety records than others, even though those hospitals do not have any more resources than the more dangerous ones. The fact is that improving safety does not require a lot of additional resources. What it requires is leadership and the will to create a culture of safety.[2]

A Culture of Safety

Five key steps are involved in building and sustaining a culture of safety, and two key issues must be confronted if the culture is to be maintained. The description below represents a simplified process which managers can tailor to the complexity of specific situations.

Make Safety a Management Priority

This should go without saying, but it is an indispensable first step toward building the culture. Safety must be in an organization's mission statement. It must be in its strategic plan. Key executives must have defined responsibilities in the area of safety. People and resources must be devoted to safety issues. An effective safety program requires a senior leader, defined program objectives, dedicated personnel, and a budget. The program must set objectives and monitor its progress by gathering data. And it must be held accountable for meeting its objectives.

Create a Learning Organization

"Learning organization," has become a buzzword, but it provides a useful description of what is required to make a safety program effective. No organization can improve its safety record, for example, if it blames individuals when adverse events occur. If they do, adverse events simply will not be reported, or they will be covered up. What is required instead is a wholly nonpunitive approach in which open communication is encouraged and accidents are responded to positively. "Let's figure out what happened here and how we can keep it from happening again" is a far more productive reaction than "Let's find out whose fault this was." The former approach leads to learning, the latter only to recrimination.

Value the Employees

It is a curious fact that the objective of the healthcare system is to take care of patients, but healthcare organizations often do not take care of their own staff. People are overworked. Staffing ratios are stretched to the limit. Many professionals—nurses in particular—do not feel valued. How can we create a safe environment for patients when nurses are subject to needle sticks, back strains, and other hazards as part of their daily work? And how can we create a safe environment when employees are treated poorly, when they are put down, shamed, or humiliated? On the positive side, think of the energy and ideas that might be tapped if employees felt valued and wanted to make a contribution. I am reminded of the story told by a former administrator of NASA (National Aeronautic Space Administration) some years ago. On one of his first days on the job, he came across a janitor sweeping the floor and asked him, "What do you do here?" The janitor replied, "We're sending a man to the moon." Suppose you could walk around a hospital and the people who sweep the floor were to tell you "We're making this the safest hospital in America."

Think in Terms of Systems

Much as we tend to blame individuals for errors, errors are rarely the result of a single blunder. Rather, they are the effect of a poorly designed system. The system may have created stresses that led to errors, or the procedures may not have been designed to be error-free. In this sense, errors are failures of management, because management did not design a better system. In other words, the causes of errors are multiple and complex; there is rarely any single cause. This is the value of conducting a root cause analysis when an error occurs. It is even more valuable if the analysis discovers accidents waiting to happen and changes the system before it produces an error.[3] The "small bites" approach to systems change—pursuing many short-cycle-time experiments (see chapter 4)—is essential.

Safety Is Everyone's Responsibility

It is difficult to change people's behavior; it takes a concerted effort. The board of trustees must provide resources and create an expectation of safety. Management must create a safe environment and take the lead in changing faulty systems. Professionals must practice safe care. Every employee must lend a hand in identifying unsafe situations. Small groups can go after small changes, try out an idea and see if it works; if it does, get more people to sign on and eventually help roll it out to the entire institution.

A few years ago, we brought 40 hospitals together at the Institute for Healthcare to form a breakthrough series collaborative, an assembly of teams from various hospitals that develop and implement best practices. The purpose of this collaborative was to reduce adverse drug events, that is, injuries related to the use or non-use of medicine. The results are reported in the *Journal of Quality Improvement*.[4] To summarize briefly, we found that some hospitals had great success and some failed. Those that did best had a firm commitment from the very top of the organization. They got all the stakeholders involved, including physicians. They set stretch goals. Interestingly, the most successful were smaller hospitals. The larger were so bureaucratic, so sclerotic, that it was very difficult for them to make changes.

In general, the hospitals that did poorly suffered from a lack of supportive leadership, lack of well-defined aims, and difficulty in defining measures and collecting data. They failed to involve stakeholders; they encountered a lot of resistance from physicians and nurses. Some broke one of the key rules: they focused on individual error, not on the system that produced the error.

Full Disclosure

Improving everyday performance is only one aspect of building a culture of safety. Another is how the hospital responds when an error is committed and results in harm to a patient. Too often, the response is a combination of denial, cover-up, and stonewalling. Don't tell the patient. Don't acknowledge anything to the family. Don't put it in the chart. Above all, don't let anything leak out to the public. The reason for covering up is the same as for cover-ups everywhere: the organization does not want to look bad, and it does not want to be sued. Of course, the information often leaks out anyway. Then the hospital or doctor frantically tries to cover their tracks while the malpractice lawyers begin sharpening their pencils.

The tragedy of all this is that most patients do not want to sue. A colleague at the Harvard School of Public Health, Leonard Marcus, is a widely known authority in the field of negotiation and conflict resolution in healthcare; he runs a program for patients who have a health-related claim and who agree to submit to mediation rather than file a suit. The patients in his program, Marcus reports, nearly all want the same things: a full and honest description of what actually happened; an apology from the people responsible, whether it is the doctor or the senior management of an institution; and an assurance that everything possible is being done to prevent the same thing from happening again. I call that full disclosure.

In an organization, full disclosure begins with a written policy enunciated by the CEO and supported by the board. The policy has to be crystal clear, and it has to be communicated effectively to the entire staff. The best disclosure policy begins from the patient's point of view and assumes that the patient wants to know everything relevant to his or her situation. The watchword here is transparency. Accumulating evidence suggests that transparency *reduces* liability risks rather than increasing them, particularly if it is coupled with a system that compensates patients when they suffer an injury from an adverse event.[5] The Veterans Administration (VA) hospitals have a policy of transparency. Hospitals that follow the VA's lead, and there are only a few of them so far, have fewer lawsuits than other hospitals.

A full disclosure policy makes it easier for physicians and other staff members to talk to patients honestly. But *how* information is disclosed is as important as the policy. Few people in this world face the physician's difficult task of telling a family that their loved one died or was injured as a result of something the physician did or did not do. It is very, very difficult to face a family and tell them what happened honestly and compassionately, when you are consumed with remorse, anguish, and shame. The point is that open, honest communication of errors is not something you just do. People need training. The apology, for instance, should not be "I'm sorry I screwed up." It should be "I'm really sorry this happened." Then the physician should go on and describe the facts, including what he or she understands about why it happened. Communication also is a team effort. Often someone else should be with the physician when he or she tells a family what happened.

The Children's Hospitals and Clinics of Minneapolis–St. Paul, Minnesota, have such a disclosure policy. The policy requires that communication be full, open, and timely. As soon as doctors know that something is really wrong, they are obligated to find out what they can about the problem, tell the patient what happened, and then tell them they are sorry and that they are looking into why it happened. The patient must receive a follow-up report within 48 hours. It is a matter of the policy that the hospital takes responsibility for adverse events, and that patients receive support when they are victims of adverse events. Several other hospitals have similar policies. The Joint Commission on Accreditation of Healthcare Organizations (JCAHO) has issued standards on disclosure, and the American Hospital Association has developed a disclosure checklist.[6] So there are many models and guidelines for full disclosure.

One last word on this subject. Full disclosure is a controversial issue. Some doctors feel that requiring full disclosure is punishment of the physician. That at least acknowledges the reality that there is no way around the difficulties physicians face when they acknowledge mistakes. But a good full disclosure policy does not put the burden entirely on physicians. The organization shares responsibility and helps the physician cope. The understanding is that errors reflect defects in a system, not simple human mistakes. In a malpractice suit, physicians often stand alone. In a good full-disclosure system, they never do.

Problem Doctors

Now and then a headline in the newspaper refers to "bad" doctors. While there probably are a few bad doctors, people who actually wish their patients harm, the real concern of a culture of safety is *problem* doctors, physicians whose performance is substandard and unsafe.

This is a rather large category. For example, about 10 percent of Americans are alcoholics, so it is safe to assume that about 10 percent of physicians are alcoholics. About 5 percent of Americans have a drug problem, and about 5 percent of physicians have a drug problem. (Doctors tend to abuse legal rather than illegal drugs, but any drug problem is a drug problem.) Ten to 20 percent of Americans at some time in their life suffer from a severe depressive episode that requires treatment. Ten to 20 percent of doctors at some time in their life are likely to suffer from a severe depressive episode that requires treatment.

Nor do these broad categories exhaust the range of problems. A small number of physicians have no simple clinical diagnosis but suffer from what might be called personality problems. They are loud, abusive, disruptive, or hostile. Another small group has not kept up their skills and are regarded by their peers as borderline incompetents. Altogether you have perhaps 25 to 30 percent of doctors who experience a serious problem at one time or another in their career and need help. These physicians should not necessarily be drummed out of the profession or lose their licenses. But if they do not get help, they will practice unsafe medicine, and eventually they will hurt somebody.

Unfortunately, organized medicine has not been good at dealing with this issue. Some states have helpful programs for dealing with alcohol and drug dependency among medical professionals but not for other problems. Hospitals and other healthcare organizations are usually very slow to react to a problem doctor. They ignore the early warning signs, and they typically do not take action until something terrible occurs. Physicians, for their part, usually find it distasteful to judge their peers. They find it emotionally difficult to condemn someone with whom they went to school or played golf, and who at the very least is a colleague laboring under the same conditions they are laboring under. Physicians also fear retribution: If we do this to him now, will they come looking for me next time around? There is seldom a good mechanism through which concerns can be expressed and those with problems can be helped.

The trouble here is much the same as the trouble with safety generally. The tendency is to blame individuals rather than the system. Think of problem doctors as part of a system and it becomes much easier to address the situation. It also becomes easier to think of a solution, which is to set up a better system to deal with the problems.

What does a system approach mean in this case? For one thing, it requires data that are missing in most healthcare organizations. For example, peers, staff, and supervisors or department chairs can routinely grade physicians. This is known in industry as a 360-degree evaluation, and it is becoming more and more commonly practiced. (Professors in many colleges and graduate programs are graded by their students, which is much the same idea.) With data gathered on everybody, not just the alleged problem doctors, leaders can identify early the people who may need help. To be sure, anyone can get an occasional negative evaluation from people with whom they just don't get along or from people with personality problems of their own. But regular, repeated evaluations from a broad range of peers and coworkers will distinguish the physician who is the object of an occasional gripe from the physician who has real problems. Another source of data can be patient complaint letters. If a doctor gets more than two a year, researchers have found, he is likely to be in one or another category of problem physicians.

Once the data have been collected, a variety of responses are possible. Often, just making physicians aware that they have a problem is sufficient. In one study, for instance, about 50 percent of physicians changed their behavior after learning that they were responsible for a disproportionate number of patient complaint letters. A second approach is to make counseling easily available, which most hospitals do not now do. An effective professional accountability system should include at least four elements: (1) performance standards, (2) mandatory compliance, (3) 360-degree evaluation, and (4) remediation programs.

Performance Standards Must Be Established

Right now, most physicians are examined for licenses and board certification just once. The aging certification parchments hang on office walls. A better approach may be a maintenance-of-certification system that would require physicians to demonstrate continuing learning and competencies. Specialty boards now are developing competency measures. Hospitals need to spell out the standards of behavior expected of physicians and other staff members: no hostile behavior, no humiliation of residents or nurses, no derogatory comments about colleagues, and so on.

Adherence to Standards Must Be a Condition of Reappointment to the Staff

Performance standards need teeth. Physicians and other professionals who cannot live up to the performance standards cannot continue working at the organization. Again, the point is not to get rid of people but to identify and help those with problems. In most cases, the threat of termination would not be invoked.

Adherence Must Be Monitored for Everyone

The use of 360-degree evaluations and other tools are a powerful sign that the organization's management takes adherence very seriously. There can be no exceptions to the rule that everyone's performance is monitored and that breaches of standards are addressed. Nothing undermines a system faster than the belief that it doesn't apply to everyone.

Remediation Programs Must Be Made Available

Finally, there should be a broad repertoire of programs for remediation. The repertoire should include psychiatric care, substance-abuse counseling, referrals to external programs or courses, and the like, as well as one-on-one reviews and informal counseling.

Bringing About Change

It may seem that creating a culture of safety is a tall order, and it is. There are many, many sources of error that need to be addressed on a system-wide basis. Organizations must learn to pursue a policy of full disclosure and to put in place all the practices that can make that policy a reality. The way organizations deal with problem doctors needs a top-to-bottom overhaul. They must move from a philosophy of identifying the bad apples to a philosophy of helping everyone to be better apples.

There are substantial rewards to making these changes, and not only because they are the right things to do. If problems that can bring an organization down—terrible errors, cover-ups, a couple of problematic doctors—are addressed, liability risks are likely to decline. The organization becomes a better place to work. It becomes a workplace characterized by mutual respect, by accountability, and by putting the patient's interest first. It becomes a workplace characterized by mutual trust. This chapter suggests several practical considerations for busy clinicians, which may encourage a culture of safety:

- Speak up for and work with leaders in your institution to create a culture where patient safety is a priority and it is safe to discuss errors.
- Demonstrate and advocate for respectful treatment of all employees and professionals.
- Actively participate in systems ("root cause") analyses of adverse events—shift the focus from the individual to the systems failure.
- Work toward developing a meaningful full-disclosure policy for patients who have experienced adverse events.
- Speak up for and help develop constructive methods for early identification and treatment of physician performance problems.

Notes

1. For a discussion on the extent of medication related errors and the benefits of employing a systems analysis when addressing this category of mistakes, see Lucian L. Leape et al., "System Analysis of Adverse Drug Events," *Journal of the American Medical Association* 274 (1995): 35–43.

2. For a general overview of the causes and extent of medical errors, as well as a set of remedial measures to create a culture and systems of safety, see Lucian L. Leape, "Error in Medicine," *Journal of the American Medical Association* 272 (1994): 1851–1857.

3. Lucian L. Leape, "Preventing Medical Accidents: Is 'Systems Analysis' the Answer?" *American Journal of Law and Medicine* 27, no. 2/3 (2001): 145–148.

4. Lucian L. Leape et al., "Reducing Adverse Drug Events: Lessons from a Breakthrough Series Collaborative," *Journal of Quality Improvement* 26 (2000): 321–331.

5. Lucian L. Leape, "Reporting Adverse Events," *The New England Journal of Medicine* 347, no. 20 (2002): 1634, 1638.

6. See "Disclosure of Unanticipated Outcomes," *Healthcare Risk Control System,* Incident Reporting and Management section, Supplement A, 5:1–13 (Plymouth Meeting, Pa.: ECRI [formerly the Emergency Care Research Institute], 2002).

6

Assessing Quality: Today's Data and a Research Agenda

CHRISTINE G. WILLIAMS

If trust in the healthcare system has eroded—and there is good evidence that it has—what are the immediate causes, the trust busters? And what can be done to rebuild trust? The U.S. Agency for Healthcare Research and Quality (AHRQ) and other organizations have sponsored research over the years to address these questions. But there are still many questions for which we have no answers, and which need to be the focus of future research. This chapter reviews the trust busters and the trust builders and addresses some of these questions.

Whatever the broad social causes of declining trust may be (see the chapters 2 and 3 by Robert Blendon and Pippa Norris, respectively), the proximate causes seem to revolve around people's experiences with the healthcare system and their perceptions of the system. The rise of for-profit healthcare organizations, for example, has led to concerns that providers put profits over patient care. So has the rise of managed care. Some states have passed patient protection laws, which may not have been necessary if patients had greater trust in managed care plans.

Another source of mistrust is inadequate communication between doctors and patients. Patients want to understand treatment alternatives and feel free to express their preferences. But research suggests that many physicians are stuck in traditional approaches. According to one study, 83 percent of physicians discuss their decisions with patients. But only 14 percent discuss alternatives; only 9 percent discuss the pros and cons of various alternatives; only 5 percent discuss the uncertainty surrounding their decisions; and only 2 percent attempt to assess the patient's understanding of the situation. Physicians in this study attempted to elicit the patient's preference only 19 percent of the time, that is, on slightly fewer than one in five occasions.[1]

Disparities in healthcare access and treatment are a source of mistrust as well. It has been well documented that African Americans and other minorities do not receive the same level of care as Caucasians, and that the poor do not receive the same level as the better off. A study sponsored by AHRQ, for example, found that slightly more than 50 percent of people who needed urgent care "always" received it, and about 30 percent "usually" received it. In this case, the figures for African Americans and Caucasians were quite similar, but they were significantly lower for Hispanics. Such disparities have percolated their way into the popular perception of how things work in healthcare. A newspaper cartoon shows an African American woman on the examining table with the doctor listening to her heart. "Give it to me straight, Doc . . . I can take it. What's wrong with me?" she asks. "You're not a white male," he replies.[2]

Sometimes perceived disparities are particularly stark. Shortly after September 11, 2001, letters containing anthrax were mailed to several members of Congress. As soon as Senate Majority Leader Tom Daschle received the letters, the Senate office building was shut down and staffers were sent home. The building was not reopened for months. When letters containing anthrax went through the Brentwood post office, however—an office staffed primarily by working-class minorities—the postal service kept the building open. The feeling among postal employees was that Senate staffers, who were mostly white and upper middle class, were being protected while they were being exposed.

Perhaps the biggest trust buster in healthcare is medical error. People's concern about this issue has peaked in recent years. In 1997, the National Patient Safety Foundation asked people, "Have you, a close friend, or a relative ever been involved in a situation where a medical mistake was made?" Some 42 percent of respondents said yes.[3] Meanwhile, press accounts of errors, often sensational, have proliferated: "Medical Error or Murder? Doctor on Trial in Baby's Death;" "Bad Reactions to Drugs Linked to Human Error;" "Fatal Goof Jolts Famous Cancer Institute;" "Injection Leaves Baby with Brain Damage." By 2000, concerns were widespread. The Kaiser Family Foundation and AHRQ asked people how concerned they were in different situations about an injury-causing medical error happening to them or their families. Nearly half said they were "very concerned" when receiving healthcare or visiting a hospital (Figure 6.1).

This is an area in which perceptions differ markedly between the general public and physicians. The public seems to welcome media accounts, even to rely on them, while physicians and hospital administrators tend to believe that the media sensationalize and exaggerate the scope of the problem. Physicians often prefer the term "patient safety" to "medical errors," which they see as a negatively loaded phrase; the public is not quite sure what patient safety means, but it knows quite well what a medical error is. Physicians do not even seem to agree with the public on the level of concern about the problem of patient safety. In a recent survey, only 29 percent of doctors thought that there were problems with the quality of healthcare in the United States. By contrast, some 68 percent of households believed that there were problems.

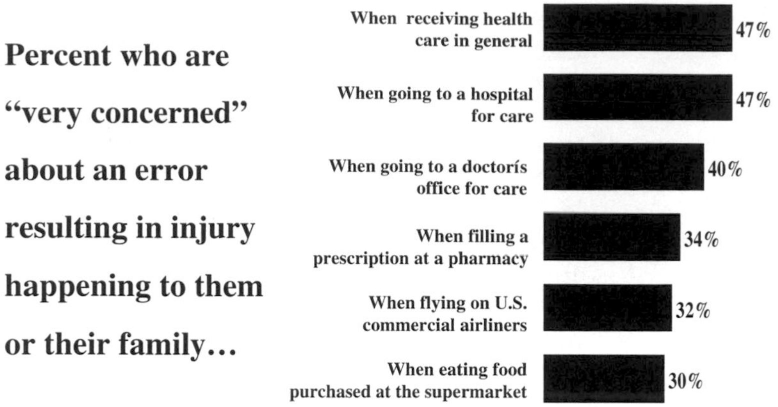

Percent who are

"very concerned"

about an error

resulting in injury

happening to them

or their family...

When receiving health care in general	47%
When going to a hospital for care	47%
When going to a doctorís office for care	40%
When filling a prescription at a pharmacy	34%
When flying on U.S. commercial airliners	32%
When eating food purchased at the supermarket	30%

Figure 6.1. Public concerns about experiencing an error

Source: Kaiser Family Foundation/Agency for Healthcare Research and Quality, National Survey on Americans as Health Care Consumers: An Update on the Role of Quality, Information, December 2000 (conducted July 31–October 13, 2000). Adapted and updated from Christine G. Williams, M.Ed., presentation at The Public's Health: A Matter of Trust Symposium, 2002, Harvard University School of Public Health.

Rebuilding Trust: Patient-Centered Care

The important trust builders in healthcare flow naturally from the nature of the trust busters. We need to address disparities in care. We need to promote and support efforts to reduce medical errors, to promote patient safety. We need a culture that takes a proactive approach to safety, rather than the "blame and shame" culture that is so common today. We need honest and extensive communication between physicians and patients and between physicians and their employers, including managed care organizations, hospitals, and other healthcare facilities. Generally, however, we need a different model of medical care, a model that puts the patient squarely in the driver's seat. We need a model in which patients and physicians are partners, or coproducers, of care.

The patient-centered care model involves patients in three ways. First, they are *decision makers.* They choose their healthcare plan, their healthcare provider, where and when to receive care, and where and when to utilize medications prescribed to them. Second, they are *participants* in their own care. They take responsibility for their choices about diet, exercise, stress, and other lifestyle behaviors that affect their health. They are involved in the management of chronic or long-term illnesses and conditions. Third, they are *evaluators* of their care. They report on their experiences and on their level of satisfaction with the entire system—physicians and other clinicians, insurers, hospitals, and so on.

What would such a model look like in practice? Imagine a woman with severe chronic obstructive pulmonary disease, or COPD. She is homebound and lives with her daughter. In the past, the woman might have been expected to get herself to the doctor's office or the medical center periodically for tests. Today, it is possible for her primary care physician to monitor her condition at home. Her daughter, for instance, might routinely e-mail peak flow measurements to the physician's practice and receive an e-mail response regarding how to adjust medication doses. Such a regimen is cheaper, easier, and more effective than the traditional approach, and it is likely to prevent her being hospitalized for COPD exacerbation. Another example of patient-centered care is the Comprehensive Health Enhancement Support System, or CHESS. This computer-based system gives people with specific conditions, such as human immunodeficiency virus infection, or HIV, access to information, advice from experts, and support from other patients. It allows patients to go through what amounts to a decision tree, helping them to make decisions about their illness and its treatment. According to AHRQ research, HIV patients using CHESS had fewer hospital admissions and incurred lower costs. They actually brought new information to their physicians about what was happening with their disease.

The patient-centered model is based on the idea that patients can get the information and learn the skills they need to be effective coproducers of care. This is no small task. It requires the comunication of customized, evidence-based information and education to patients on a regular basis. Care must be coordinated and integrated, so that they do not hear one thing from one doctor and something entirely different from another. Healthcare providers must learn to share decision making with patients and their families, and patients must learn the skills involved in managing their own care. Electronic communication is essential to the entire enterprise. Patients need access to Web-based applications and self-management programs such as CHESS. Physicians and hospitals must learn to communicate electronically with patients and vice versa.

Can patients truly evaluate the care they receive? To answer this question fairly, two measures of performance, clinical quality, and patient satisfaction, must be looked at separately. Often the issue of evaluation focuses on clinical quality, and though patients may have a greater role to play in assessing clinical quality in the future, that role will always be somewhat limited by their lack of professional knowledge and experience. Patient satisfaction is another matter entirely. No one can judge that as well as patients themselves. Moreover, satisfaction is undoubtedly as important as clinical quality. Patients who are more satisfied are more likely to comply with treatment regimens, more likely to provide relevant information to their healthcare provider, more likely to return for care, and more likely to experience better outcomes. It is obviously a critical measure, if we care about rebuilding trust in the healthcare system.

One of the most ambitious efforts to assess patient experiences of care is AHRQ's Consumer Assessment of Health Plans (CAHPs), a kit of survey and report tools that provides reliable and valid information to help consumers and purchasers assess and choose among health plans. The purpose of CAHPs is to gather information about the quality of people's experience in healthcare, particularly with health plans. Interestingly, the first annual report from the National CAHPs Benchmarking Database found that plan enrollees rate their healthcare highly. They report largely positive experiences with providers and staff. There are differences in ratings and reports among various groups—commercial plans, Medicaid, and Medicare—with Medicare enrollees reporting the most positive experiences. (Some speculate that this may be because people over 65 are more likely to accept what their physicians are telling them. When the baby boomers hit 65 and go on Medicare, they may be more likely to challenge their healthcare providers.) CAHPs include questions about specific experiences of patients and consumers. Did they have a problem getting a referral to a specialist? Did they feel that doctors and other providers were listening carefully to them? Were there any problems with the customer service or the paperwork required by the health plan?

The potential of this kind of research has not yet been realized. Ultimately, consumers may use the data to evaluate their own experiences against those of others and to make smarter decisions about health plans and providers. Health plans and providers can use the data to evaluate their own performance and to map areas that need improvement. The entire enterprise can be a powerful tool for quality improvement.

A Research Agenda

Any review of trust busters and potential trust builders raises more questions than it can hope to answer. We do not yet know enough about assessing and improving healthcare performance or how patients can play an effective role in their own care. In particular, we need a research agenda that addresses issues such as consumer education, development of standardized measures, alignment of issues, and the relationship between healthcare performance and trust.

Consumer Education

Many believe that consumer education has great potential to improve the quality of healthcare. But how can effective consumer education programs be implemented? They cannot be one-shot deals; they must be sustained over time and repeated as necessary. And they must be evaluated at every step to ensure that they are achieving the intended objectives.

Development of Standardized Measures

The only way to assess healthcare performance accurately is to compare apples to apples, that is, to use standardized measures. What measures have proved to be useful? What other measures are needed? What are the best ways to develop them? How can measures be used to encourage continuous improvement?

The Alignment of Incentives

The market offers healthcare providers a variety of incentives, some of them contradictory. We need to study how incentives from the market, from regulators, and from organizational purchasing policies can be used to push improvements in quality.

The Relationship between Healthcare Performance and Trust

Everybody agrees that rebuilding trust is critical to patient satisfaction. But what are the most effective avenues to greater trust? Does public reporting of performance measures increase trust or undermine it? Some physicians and hospitals appear to be uncomfortable with information being reported to the public, yet consumer organizations indicate that they want more information. Then, too, how does trust relate to expectations? Medicare enrollees, as suggested earlier, may be more satisfied with the healthcare system simply because they have lower expectations. Ultimately, questions about the nature of trust need to be examined. Can trust be quantified? Is it a good in itself or a means to an end? Does it have a positive effect on an organization's bottom line?

The potential of research to affect cost, access, and quality of healthcare is significant. Take one example, benign prostatic hyperplasia, or BPH. In the past, most men with BPH underwent surgery to correct this condition, and too often patients became impotent or incontinent as a result. Eventually, studies showed that surgery was not always advisable. The condition in some cases could be treated by new medications and in other cases did not need to be treated immediately at all (watchful waiting). The number of operations declined by 50 percent over the last decade, and patients learned to play an active role in shared decision making. This is the kind of improvement that can be hoped for in other areas—better information, better outcomes, and ultimately greater trust.

The Doctor-Patient Relationship

What can busy clinicians do to overcome the problem of trust in the healthcare system? While physicians and other clinicians do not have control over every component of the system, they are the primary contact for patients. An improved trust relationship between patients and clinicians is the starting point for overall improvement throughout the healthcare system.

First, clinicians must communicate openly and honestly with their patients. They should encourage their patients to ask questions and make sure they understand the answers. Clinicians should speak honestly and share with patients both the uncertainty about and the options for treatment.

Second, physicians and other clinicians must treat patients and their families as partners in their healthcare. Even a busy physician's office can provide information to patients through print, video or online resources, so that the patient begins to understand his condition and the need to be a partner in his care. Physicians may be able to provide shared decision-making tools for patients and families or help patients with chronic diseases enroll in self-management programs.

Third, clinicians may be able to enhance communication with their patients through e-mail or other electronic methods. An investment in these communications methods may result in fewer office visits and improved trust between clinicians and patients.

Finally, clinicians must work with others in the healthcare system to improve trust with patients. Clinicians can involve nurses and other members of an office practice to improve support for and communication with patients. Clinicians must build effective teams within office practices as well as larger systems of care, if trust in the healthcare system is to improve.

Notes

1. Clarence H. Braddock, Stephan D. Fihn, Wendy Levinson, Albert R. Jonsen, and Robert A. Pearlman, "How Doctors and Patients Discuss Routine Clinical Decisions: Informed Decision Making in the Outpatient Setting," *Journal of General Internal Medicine* 12 (1997): 339–345.

2. As cited in the meeting transcript of the Department of Health and Human Services, National Committee on Vital and Health Statistics, Subcommittee on Populations, February 11, 2002. Available: http://www.ncvhs.hhs.gov/020211tr.htm (accessed April 5, 2006).

3. Louis Harris & Associates, "Public Opinion of Patient Safety Issues: Research Findings," prepared for the National Patient Safety Foundation (September 1997), 34.

III

Who Can Be Trusted?

7

Patients' Trust in Their Doctors:
Are We Losing Ground?

DANA GELB SAFRAN

What does it mean to say a patient has trust in his or her doctor? My colleagues and I have used a three-part definition of trust in our research into the doctor-patient relationship, a definition that has guided our approach to measuring trust. In this definition, patient trust is characterized by:

- Confidence in the doctor's *integrity*. The patient believes that the doctor is honest and truthful, and that the doctor will keep the patient's information confidential. The patient also believes that the doctor will communicate openly, even if he or she makes a mistake.
- Confidence in the doctor's *clinical knowledge and skill*. The patient believes that the doctor has the technical knowledge needed to provide effective treatment, that the doctor's skills are up-to-date, and that the doctor will know when additional treatment or specialty care is necessary.
- Confidence in the doctor as the *patient's fiduciary agent*. The patient believes that the doctor's treatment recommendations are based solely and entirely on consideration of what is in the patient's best interest and are not based on the best interests of other parties (e.g., the patient's health plan, the physician's practice, the physician's financial interest).

Thinking about trust in these terms, it is perhaps easy to see why it has become a topic of widespread interest in recent years and why it is likely to remain so in the future. Patients today continue to express high levels of trust and confidence in their physicians. But changes in healthcare delivery, including changes in how physicians are paid and in the autonomy they exercise over treatment decisions, have put the third element of trust—patients' confidence in the doctor as their agent—in some jeopardy. Patients have begun to wonder: When my doctor confers with my insurance company before making a treatment decision, how are they deciding whether to do that test for me or offer that procedure to me? Does my doctor have financial incentives that I don't know about? An influential article published a few years ago refers to physicians as "double agents," pointing to their dual role as actors entrusted by patients and by organizations such as health plans, with both parties expecting the physician to do no harm to their best interests.[1] It is often a precarious balancing act, and as patients have become aware of this, many have become concerned.

Today, many features of managed care that put physicians in this dual role are subsiding, and as they do, concerns about fiduciary trust should ease. In place of this issue, however, I believe there looms an even more pervasive challenge to one of the three elements of patient trust, namely confidence in the physician's technical knowledge and skill. In the information age, the abundance of online medical advice and patients' use of this information presents a new challenge to the doctor-patient relationship. We do not yet have empirical studies of the impact on trust, but the anecdotal evidence is abundant. Physicians report that patients come to their offices with a lot of information (and misinformation) obtained from the Internet and with opinions about possible courses of treatment.[2] Some express these opinions vociferously and then feel a lack of trust if the doctor does not readily go along. At a minimum, this can set up a difficult dynamic between doctor and patient, particularly if the doctor is feeling pressed for time and is unable to fully discuss the information with the patient. In some cases, physicians resent being put in a position of having their medical judgment second-guessed by the Internet and respond negatively. The potential in these situations for strain on the doctor-patient relationship, and on patient trust, is clear.

In addition, some patients feel reticent to express their opinions and come to the office with a clear expectation of what the physician ought to do in response to the health problem they are presenting. For example, information gotten from a Web site or a television advertisement may have persuaded the patient that a particular medication would dramatically improve their chronic acid reflux condition. When the doctor fails to prescribe that medication, and the patient fails to ask about it, the patient may walk away with a nagging doubt as to whether the doctor really knows the latest in medical treatments for his condition. The challenges to the doctor-patient relationship—particularly patient trust—that have arrived with the information age are likely to be longlasting and must be addressed to avoid a negative downward spiral in the quality of doctor-patient interactions.

There is another powerful reason for studying trust in the doctor-patient relationship right now: morale among physicians has been never been lower than it is today. Here is a sampling of comments from primary care physicians in Massachusetts from a survey conducted in 2001:

- "I don't know how much longer I can hold on. I keep hoping there'll be a turnaround, but it doesn't seem to be coming."
- "I can't think of a colleague that has a positive view of the current practice environment."
- "It is terrible. Fragmented, obstructed, restricted, demoralizing—emphasis totally on the bottom line, the institutions are crippled."

A longitudinal study of primary care physicians in Massachusetts assessed several different measures of morale in 1986 and again in 1997. The measures included physicians' opinions as to the quality of healthcare they were providing, the time they were able to spend with patients, their autonomy, their leisure time, and their earnings. All of these declined over the 11-year period, and for several elements of physician satisfaction, the decline was significant. Moreover, the 1996 scores were startlingly low. Only 36 percent of physicians were "satisfied" or "very satisfied" with the incentives to provide high-quality care in their practice; only 42 percent were satisfied or very satisfied with the amount of time they were able to spend with patients. Sixty percent were satisfied or very satisfied with their degree of autonomy, down from 75 percent in 1986. The only measure that still ranked high was satisfaction with the quality of care they were able to provide—91 percent in 1997, down from 98 percent in 1986.[3]

In light of such data it may be useful to try to untangle the doctor-patient relationship, particularly the relationship between primary care physicians and their patients. This is one key point at which trust in healthcare can be built or undermined.

Assessing the Primary Care Relationship

About ten years ago, the Institute of Medicine (IOM) defined primary care as follows: "Primary care is the provision of integrated, accessible healthcare services by clinicians who are accountable for addressing a large majority of personal health needs, developing a sustained partnership with patients, and practicing in the context of family and community."[4] Note a couple of salient phrases in this definition, neither of which appeared in an earlier (1978) definition. One is "sustained partnership." Continuity had always been seen as essential to primary care. But some had come to interpret this as achievable through the medical record. With the phrase "sustained partnership," the IOM made explicit that primary care is predicated on continuity between human beings. The other notable change was the use of the phrase "practicing in the context of family and community." Earlier definitions had always underscored that primary care required a comprehensive approach, but the IOM made explicit that primary care is unique in emphasizing a whole-person orientation to care rather than focusing on a particular disease or organ system. Through its definition, the IOM underscored that primary care requires both knowing patients' medical situations and knowing their life circumstances.

The IOM's definition, of course, is formal. But if you ask physicians to define primary care, what you hear is not so different. One said, "Other men and women are responsible for different parts and pieces and different areas," but there must be, there has to be, there should be one person responsible for the whole picture. [Someone] who has the ability, cognitively and emotionally, to put it all together and to put the different recommendations into the context of that patient's life." Said another, "The other piece of continuous care is that it's a commitment to the patient that you are going to be there tomorrow and the next day. That what you do now is going to be building for everything you're going to be doing in the future."

And yet another said, "You'll be the one to make the diagnosis, to decide if they need to see any specialists for further evaluation, and then, you'll be the person, if you're doing your job right, who will pull it all together, who will counsel the person around all the different opinions and help guide them through what has to be done. It's really first, middle and last."[5] Like the IOM, these physicians see themselves as treating the whole patient. The primary care relationship is at the center, with other medical systems around it to be called upon as needed.

Over a ten-year period of research, my colleagues and I developed and validated a set of measures to assess this relationship. The Primary Care Assessment Survey (PCAS) is a brief, patient-completed questionnaire that measures each of the defining characteristics outlined by the IOM's definition of primary care. The measures have been extensively tested and validated; all scales exceed established standards for excellent instrumentation and perform consistently well across population subgroups defined according to patient sociodemographics and health status. The PCAS measures cover seven defining characteristics of primary care with 11 summary scales, as follows: access to care (organizational, financial), continuity (longitudinal, visit-based), comprehensiveness of care (knowledge of patient, preventive counseling), integration of care, clinical interaction (clinician-patient communication, thoroughness of physical examinations), interpersonal treatment, and trust. Thus, the PCAS measures provide a richly detailed view of the quality of the primary care relationship, as well as of patients' experiences with other important aspects of primary care such as access, continuity, and integration of care.

The first large-scale study to use the PCAS included about 6,000 adults in Massachusetts. The patients were distributed across 12 different health plans, which fell into five different models of health insurance. These models included traditional fee-for-service insurance, point-of-service insurance, network- and IPA-model HMOs, group-model HMOs, and staff-model HMOs. The study found that the highest level of performance was in the fee-for-service system and the lowest in staff model HMOs.[6] For the most part, performance declined as you moved from more "open" models, such as fee for service, to more "closed" models, such as group and staff HMOs. A second, broader study focused on a nationwide sample of Medicare recipients and compared those who were in traditional Medicare arrangements with those enrolled in Medicare HMOs. These results were consistent with the Massachusetts study: Conventional Medicare performed better across the board than managed Medicare, and within managed Medicare, open-model plans outperformed closed-model plans.[7] The quality of the doctor-patient relationship appears to be consistently stronger in open-model arrangements and in the fee-for-service system than it is in closed-model arrangements, such as the staff model HMO.

Why should this be? One theory suggests that the patient's sense of connection to the doctor, the feeling that "this is *my* doctor" is a factor. One way to build that sense of connection is through visit-based continuity; after all, it is difficult to build when the patient is seeing someone else—especially if he or she does not feel connected to these other clinicians and does not relate to them as part of the primary care team. Our studies find that patients in closed-model systems see their doctors (as opposed to another clinician in the practice) substantially less often than patients in open-model systems. Patients were asked to rate their experiences of this, and the ratings underscored that patients value continuity. Patients who were seeing their own doctor nearly all the time rated their experience as excellent. Patients who were seeing their doctor only occasionally or almost never rated their experiences as poor.

What does this imply about the potential for employing a team approach to primary care? Do practices that rely on a team approach to primary care consign patients to feeling disenfranchised from their physician and dissatisfied with their care? I do not think so. However, practices that rely on primary care teams must dedicate themselves to creating visible-team care. A visible team is one in which the individual team members and their respective roles and responsibilities are known and accepted by the patient. This is contrasted with invisible-team care, in which the patient is unclear about who will be involved in their care at the practice, how these clinicians relate to each other, and what role each plays in their care. The invisible-team care experience, from the patient's perspective, is one of interpersonal chaos and disconnection. Patients relate to other clinicians in the practice as "not my doctor" rather than as "a member of my primary care team."

Data from our research suggests that primary healthcare practices nationwide rely extensively on teams. Approximately half of patients in most care settings— and more in some settings—report that other doctors and nurses play an important role in their care. For the most part, however, patients appear to experience these other clinicians as part of an invisible team, individuals who have no particular knowledge about them or connection to them but who provide care when their doctor is not available. This was the case in primary care practices nationwide, even those in closed-model systems, which are typically designed around a team approach. Reflecting on the IOM definition of primary care, particularly the notion that primary care requires sustained partnerships and a whole-person orientation to care, data from patients underscore that we have a long way to go to realize this through our use of primary care teams.

Outcomes: The Role of Trust

The ultimate reason for evaluating and monitoring the quality of the doctor-patient relationship is to improve outcomes of care. There are many types of relevant outcomes, of course. In our research, we have evaluated the role of doctor-patient relationship quality as a factor influencing two broad categories of outcomes: business outcomes and health outcomes. Business outcomes include variables such as patients' loyalty to the practice and patients' willingness to recommend the practice to family and friends. Health outcomes include variables such as whether the patient decides to follow the doctor's advice and whether their health shows measurable improvement. Ideally, we would like to find factors that improve results in both categories.

Consider the issue of loyalty to a doctor's practice. A practice with high rates of voluntary disenrollment—that is, a large percentage of patients choosing to leave the practice to obtain care elsewhere—would suggest that something is not working. But what is it and why? In principle, patients could be leaving because they are dissatisfied with their access to the physician or for other structural reasons. They also could be leaving because they are dissatisfied with the quality of their interactions with the physician. In the Massachusetts study described earlier, about 20 percent of patients left their primary physician over a three-year period. We analyzed the data to determine which factors were most important in these departure decisions.[8]

Not surprisingly, both organizational and interpersonal factors were important. But the quality of the doctor-patient relationship was considerably more important than any other factor. In fact, after accounting for differences in patient characteristics and structural variables (such as access and continuity of care), people with the poorest quality relationships with their doctor voluntarily left their doctor's practice at rates that were three times higher than those with the highest quality relationships. Of the variables defining relationship quality, moreover, the most important were trust and a whole-person orientation to care (Figure 7.1). Over a three-year study period, 37 percent of patients who began the study in the bottom 5 percent of the trust scale left their physicians, while only 11 percent of patients in the top 5 percent left theirs. The importance of relationship quality as a driver of patient retention in a practice suggests the business case for practices attending to this aspect of care.

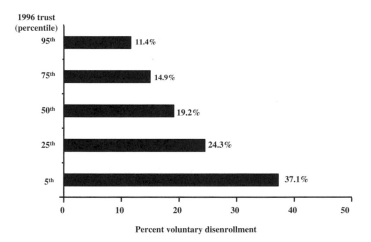

Figure 7.1. Relationship between trust and disenrollment

Source: Dana Gelb Safran et al., *Journal of Family Practice* 50 (2001): 130–136. Adapted and updated from Dana Gelb Safran, Sc.D., presentation at The Public's Health: A Matter of Trust Symposium, 2002, Harvard University School of Public Health.

The fact that relationship quality surpassed all other measures, including access to care, as a predictor of patient loyalty suggests that focusing on fast, easy appointment access is not enough. Attention to the quality of clinician-patient interactions and the establishment of high-quality primary care relationships matter more with respect to earning patients' loyalty to the practice.

A similarly strong relationship exists between trust and the patient's adherence to the doctor's advice. Adherence is a particularly important aspect of healthcare. In some cases, adherence involves patients' taking a medication that the doctor has prescribed. In other cases, adherence means changing behaviors that pose a long-term health risk, such as giving up smoking, cutting down on alcohol, or getting more exercise. These types of lifestyle changes are often extremely difficult to achieve and even more difficult to sustain. Using data from several longitudinal studies, my colleagues and I have examined the role of doctor-patient relationship quality in determining patients' adherence to their doctor's advice. In one such study, we examined the extent to which the quality of the relationship predicted patients' *attempts* to make behavior changes that their doctor had recommended; then we examined the extent to which relationship quality predicted *success* in making these changes.

We found that a large percentage of patients in our study attempted to change their behavior after being counseled by their primary physician. For example, 86 percent of smokers whose primary care doctor advised them to quit attempted to do so, and 80 percent of sedentary patients who were advised to exercise more attempted to make this change. Not surprisingly, a far smaller percentage of patients succeeded in making these behavior changes. Only 28 percent actually did give up smoking, and only 40 percent actually increased their exercise. However, the quality of the doctor-patient relationships—and trust in particular—were important predictors of both attempts to change behaviors and of success (Figure 7.2).[9] Thus, higher levels of patient trust translate into hundreds of patients in a given practice who may succeed in changing behaviors such as quitting smoking that will improve their health now and over the long term.

So the good news about trust is that it matters. Physicians can assume that successful efforts to rebuild trust among patients will have payoffs, both from a business point of view and from a medical point of view. The more discouraging news is that there is evidence that the quality of physician-patient interactions is declining and that trust is declining with it. In the national Medicare study, covering 1998 to 2000, there were significant declines in the quality of communication, interpersonal treatment and the thoroughness of physical exams.[10] Interestingly, trust did not change significantly in the elderly population over that period. However, in the Massachusetts study, covering 1996 to 1999, a significant decline in multiple aspects of the doctor-patient relationship, including trust, was observed.[11] When we analyzed the individual components of the trust scale, the biggest single drop was in patients' trust in their physician as a fiduciary agent (i.e., whether the doctor cares more about holding down costs than about patients' health. [Figure 7.3]).

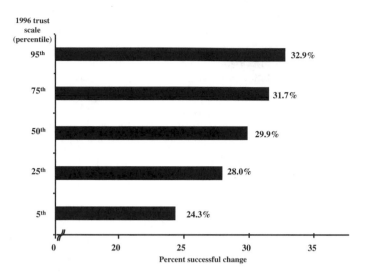

Figure 7.2. Patient trust as a predictor of adherence: Successful behavior change

Source: Dana Gelb Safran et al., *Journal of General Internal Medicine* 15, suppl. (2000): 116. Adapted and updated from Dana Gelb Safran, Sc.D., presentation at The Public's Health: A Matter of Trust Symposium, 2002, Harvard University School of Public Health.

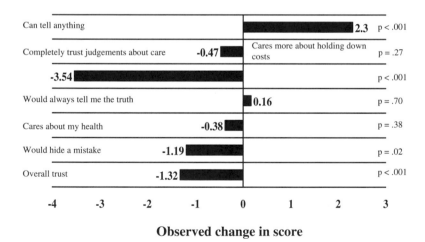

Observed change in score

Figure 7.3. Items comparing trust scale, 1996–1999

Source: J. Murphy et al., "The Quality of Physician-Patient Relationships: Patients' Experiences 1996–1999," *Journal of Family Practice* 50, no. 2 (2001): 123–129. Adapted and updated from Dana Gelb Safran, Sc.D., presentation at The Public's Health: A Matter of Trust Symposium, 2002, Harvard University School of Public Health.

Trust can be reinforced and rebuilt, though a detailed discussion of how to do so is beyond the scope of this chapter. One key ingredient, though, is for physicians and healthcare organizations to recognize that trust and the interpersonal quality of care remain at the heart of medical care and to begin to include these in our nation's portfolio of quality measures. Physicians know intuitively and empirical data show that the quality of clinician-patient relationships matters in terms of both business and health outcomes. Without our focused attention, we are losing ground. This downward slide in interpersonal quality stands in marked contrast to other areas of healthcare quality that have received focused attention through measurement and reporting and that have responded with noteworthy improvements. For example, as national quality initiatives have shined a light on rates of preventive screening, such as mammography, childhood immunizations, and good diabetic management, we have seen meaningful and impressive improvements in each of these areas.

To this point, however, the quality of physician-patient relationships and patient trust have not been part of what is routinely monitored and addressed. In the absence of this focus, and given the tremendous competing priorities and time pressures, the downward trend in physician-patient relationship quality seen in both local and national studies can be expected to continue. To reverse this trend will require that practices and healthcare organizations dedicate themselves to this important feature of healthcare quality as well as to many others. The benefits of doing so will accrue to patients, to the physicians who care for them, and to the practices in which they work.

Notes

1. Stephen M. Shortell et al., "Physicians as Double Agents: Maintaining Trust in an Era of Multiple Accountabilities," *Journal of the American Medical Association* 280 (1998): 1102–1108.

2. Elizabeth Murray et al., "The Impact of Health information on the Internet on Health Care and the Physician-Patient Relationship: National U.S. Survey on 1,050 U.S. Physicians," *Journal of Medical Internet Research* 5 (2005): e17.

3. Alison Murray et al., "Doctor Discontent: A Comparison of Physician Satisfaction in Different Delivery System Settings, 1986 and 1997," *Journal of General Internal Medicine* 16 (2001): 451–459.

4. Institute of Medicine, *Primary Care: America's Health in a New Era* (Washington, DC: National Academy Press, 1996).

5. D. G. Safran, "Defining the Future of Primary Care: What Can We Learn from Patients?" *Annals of Internal Medicine* 138 (2003): 248–255.

6. D. G. Safran et al., "Organizational and Financial Characteristics of Health Plans: Are They Related to Primary Care Performance?" *Archives of Internal Medicine* 160 (2000): 69–76.

7. D. G. Safran et al., "Primary Care Quality in the Medicare Program: Comparing the Performance of Medicare Health Maintenance Organizations and Traditional Fee-for-Service Medicare," *Archives of Internal Medicine* 162 (2002): 757–765; J. E. Montgomery et al., "Primary Care Experiences of Medicare Beneficiaries, 1998–2000," *Journal of General Internal Medicine* 19 (2004): 1064–1065.

8. D. G. Safran et al., "Switching Doctors: Predictors of Voluntary Disenrollment from a Primary Physician's Practice," *Journal of Family Practice* 50 (2001): 130–136.

9. D. G. Safran et al, "Linking Doctor-Patient Relationship Quality to Outcomes," *Journal of General Internal Medicine* 15, suppl. (2000): 116.

10. D. G. Safran, "Defining the Future of Primary Care: What Can We Learn from Patients?" *Annals of Internal Medicine* 138 (2003): 248–255.

11. J. Murphy et al., "The Quality of Physician-Patient Relationships: Patients' Experiences 1996–1999," *Journal of Family Practice* 50 (2001): 123–129.

8

Healthcare Research: Can Patients Trust Physician Scientists?

GREG KOSKI

Not long ago, a *Time* magazine cover portrayed a woman in a cage with the caption "Human Guinea Pigs." Inside, readers were invited to ponder a disquieting question: "Some patients join clinical trials out of desperation, others to help medicine advance. Who is to blame if they get sick—or even die?" Behind the question lurked an even more disquieting message. Medical research is dangerous. Can you trust the doctors who are conducting it? The article continued, "Clinical trials are usually pretty safe. The vast majority of subjects are not hurt in any way. But so many problems—and such serious problems—have surfaced in recent years that doctors and hospital administrators are starting to wonder whether there is something dangerously wrong with the clinical-trial system."[1]

The *Time* article is an example of a major cause for concern—the erosion of public trust in health research. It goes without saying that progress in medicine depends greatly on research that utilizes human subjects. No one can know with certainty whether a drug or a device is safe and effective until it has been extensively tested in people. It also goes without saying that such research depends greatly on trust between the subjects of the experiment and the physician scientists who are conducting it. Without trust, the supply of volunteers for clinical trials will simply dry up, and progress in biomedical research will grind to a halt.

So what is to be done? In this chapter, I analyze some of the causes and consequences of the decline in trust and propose some cures. But it may help to first discuss some philosophical propositions that underlie our commitment to research and that show just how important trust is to the whole endeavor.

Scientific Research and Risk

Science seeks knowledge through research, and that knowledge must be based on truth. Truth is the very foundation of our trust in knowledge; we have confidence in research findings because we believe they accurately describe the way the world works. What happens when that confidence is shaken, say, because the research is exposed as flawed or fraudulent? Suddenly the knowledge ostensibly acquired by science is not only worthless, it is actually harmful. Worse, it is not just one experiment that is now subject to doubt, it is the entire scientific enterprise. If one researcher cannot be trusted, why trust the others?

Another way of understanding this point relies not on objective notions of truth or falsehood but on the very human traits of integrity and responsibility. Science, after all, is a human endeavor, conducted by human beings. We depend on these human beings to carry out their responsibilities in ways that support trust and truth. We expect both the individuals and the organizations involved in research to act with integrity and to conduct themselves responsibly. Of course, most do. The trouble is that a few do not. A single act of irresponsible conduct has ramifications that extend well beyond the boundary of any single experiment. It is in effect a body blow to the core of science because it undermines trust.

Research into health presents special problems. The goal of the research, naturally, is to improve health, to help people live longer, better lives. Nearly everybody accepts the idea that research is critically important in achieving this goal. But conducting health-related experiments nearly always involves knowingly exposing people to risk. So, protection from unnecessary risk must be an intrinsic part of the science. We cannot eliminate risk, but we can build appropriate safeguards into the methodologies that we employ to conduct the science.

Again, it helps to view this idea from a slightly different angle. One might argue that human research is inherently unethical. Immanuel Kant and many other philosophers have told us that no individual should ever be used as a means to an end. Most people agree. Yet that is precisely what human research does. Some individuals become the subjects of experimentation so that scientists can acquire knowledge and society can reap the benefits, while the individuals bearing the risk often gain nothing. We justify this conduct on the basis of utilitarianism. We say (and believe) that the research will ultimately help a larger number of people. But the inherently unethical nature of the research demands a strong moral covenant between researchers and their subjects.

Ethical Conduct and Material Gain

The research process has to be governed by ethical principles and conduct. Everyone involved has to understand that unethical conduct violates the trust that is the foundation of the research. To move from a philosophical plane to a materialistic one, it is worth noting that science does not operate in a vacuum. Drugs, devices, and biologics may indeed improve health. Those same drugs, devices, and biologics may also become patented products with huge commercial value. So there is a lot of money at stake. It is how our system operates, and it operates quite well. Yet, large amounts of money can have powerful effects on human behavior. Like most human beings, researchers are responsive to financial incentives. So, too, are the patients who are the subjects or potential subjects of the research. Companies, universities, and medical centers all respond to financial inducements as well. When pondering the possibilities for unethical behavior or behavior that generates mistrust, we would be wise not to ignore the pull of the material world.

A Legacy of Mistrust

So health research utilizing human subjects has built-in tensions. The history of this research and of the protection of subjects that it necessarily entails is not particularly encouraging either. In fact, the abuses of the past have left behind a broad legacy of mistrust. In the modern era, the seminal event of this history was the well-known 1966 article by Henry K. Beecher entitled "Ethics and Clinical Research."[2] Beecher examined some 150 examples of human-subjects research just by looking through journals on his desk. Of these, he found many that were not being conducted responsibly. Some posed serious risks to their subjects. Others had neglected to obtain informed consent. What were significant here, however, were not just Beecher's revelations but also the reactions of the research community. Rather than asking how this could happen, many researchers essentially denied that there was a problem. When the possibility of regulation arose, the research community did not welcome it.

Protection through Government Regulation

A regulatory framework intended to protect human subjects was imposed upon researchers by the government in an attempt to ensure ethical conduct by mandate. This action alone reinforced a perception that the scientific community could not be trusted to act responsibly in the absence of a legal requirement to do so.

Regrettably, the commitment of both the government and the research community to effective implementation of the regulations fell short of what was needed for success. This had serious consequences. Consider Duke University School of Medicine, which in the last 30 years became a leader in clinical research. Research is at the very core of its academic mission. Yet when government regulators investigated Duke's program in 1998, they found that the organization allocated no more than a part of one person's time to the process of protecting human subjects. This was found to be more or less standard operating procedure for many such institutions around the country. It was not that Duke administrators or anybody else were bad people. They just had many conflicting priorities and not enough resources to go around. Regulations designed to protect human subjects were viewed as one more burden rather than as an integral part of the scientific endeavor. This was a major failure of the research community.

There were failures at the government level as well. As far back as the early 1950s, the director of the National Institutes of Health (NIH) called for a system of peer review, thereby implying that the researchers could not be trusted to make good decisions without oversight. That attitude of mistrust continued for many years and culminated in the passage of the 1974 National Research Act. The act requires that organizations sponsoring research establish so-called institutional review boards (IRBs) to monitor federally funded research, and it established a federal agency (now known as the Office for Human Research Protections) to oversee the IRBs. But the government was imposing regulations on the research community without providing the necessary resources and support to aid researchers and institutions in following and implementing the regulations. It was an unfunded federal mandate. Nor were the regulations presented and interpreted in a way that helped people understand them.

At the time, most research involving human subjects was done in academic medical centers and funded by NIH. That system grew as NIH's funding grew, and IRBs did their best to take on the legacy of mistrust that had plagued the research. But during the 1980s and 1990s, more and more trials moved from academic settings to private physicians' offices, as industry became the major funding sources of human research in clinical trials. The trials could be accomplished quicker and more easily; the IRBs, if indeed there were IRBs, were more efficient and more cooperative. But the result of this shift was not always conducive to building trust. To take a hypothetical example, a patient might come to see his doctor and report that the blood pressure medication he had taken for 15 years was working fine. But the physician might say, "You know, there's a new drug coming out that perhaps you ought to try," and proceed to enroll the patient in a clinical trial. Yet the patient would not necessarily know that his doctor was an investigator working for a pharmaceutical company helping to develop that new drug. When patients learned the truth, they were rarely happy, and their trust in their physician evaporated.

In the 1980s, people in the research community began to believe that U.S. academic institutions were losing a competitive advantage in the world. They were not patenting the discoveries being made with federal support, nor were they developing those discoveries into commercial products. A movement arose to create partnerships between business and academia, with the objective of moving more discoveries into the commercial arena. Billions of industry dollars infused the research process, creating the potential for (and often the reality of) major conflicts of interest.[3] The IRBs, meanwhile, found themselves facing a vastly expanded research landscape. They had to labor mightily to carry out both their regulatory obligations and their ethical responsibilities to protect human subjects. They became the focus of frustrated scientists and sponsors eager to move their studies forward. To say that the IRBs were beleaguered and embattled would not be an overstatement.

All this took place in the context of a massive cultural change in the worlds of science and health care. Men had dominated both worlds, like they dominated the rest of society. Suddenly, women were asserting their interests and challenging the dominant paternalist culture. In a very short span of time, government policies regarding clinical trials went from excluding women, on the ground that women had to be protected, to making a point of including them, because to do otherwise would be discriminatory. Both science and health had also been dominated by an ethic that said the professionals know best. Suddenly, consumer movements were challenging that ethic. Consumers and patients were no longer willing to let someone else make decisions for them. Just as they wanted all the information they could get when they bought a new car or television set, they wanted all the information they could get about clinical trials, and they refused to participate if they did not get it. Finally, the rise of managed care dramatically changed the entire doctor-patient relationship. In principle, managed care was a fine idea, the ultimate in data-driven healthcare. In practice, however, money too often took the driver's seat, rather than the well-being of patients. Many physicians were offered incentives *not* to provide care. This often had a negative impact both on medical care and on medical research, simply because it undermined the trust that had once inhered in the doctor-patient relationship.

The cumulative result of these changes was declining confidence in the integrity of science and medicine. Scientists themselves often failed to help their cause; even the most prestigious among them sometimes seemed more concerned with financial rewards and personal advancement than with academic accomplishment. In 1999, as is well known, a young man named Jesse Gelsinger died in a clinical trial at the University of Pennsylvania. People were horrified, but it seemed at least that everything had been done right. Later, the public learned that everything had not been done right and that the principal investigator held a stake in the company that owned the rights to the drug being used in the trial. The resultant loss of trust has affected the entire research community. The mantra today is "Do it right or not at all."

Today's System and the Principles of Change

Two pillars of support for the research system, both created with the best of intentions, have evolved over the last 30 years. One is the IRBs, groups of lay people and scientists charged with reviewing human-subject research to determine whether a study is ethical and safe before approving it. The other is the process of informed consent, in which researchers are required to explain to patients what their participation in the research will involve, and what risks and benefits, if any, it may entail. Without informed consent, the research may not go forward, even though many have questioned the effectiveness of the consent procedure, which now is focused more on paperwork than on process.

Because of the way the system has been implemented, many in the research community have come to view IRBs and consent not as twin pillars but as twin barriers. Some researchers get around them or live up to the letter of the law without living up to its spirit. In 1998, the Department of Health and Human Services' Office of the Inspector General (OIG) bluntly declared that the national system for protection of research subjects was not prepared to meet the challenges of the modern research environment. The IRBs in particular were overburdened, it said, and reliance upon them to protect human research subjects was no longer an effective strategy. Interestingly, the OIG's report also declared that IRBs were the *only* bodies with the primary responsibility of protecting human subjects.[4] By implication, the report was saying that it was not the responsibility of the investigators to protect their subjects. With such an approach, it is hardly surprising that we wound up with a dysfunctional system. Nor was it surprising that the research community and government officials began to explore the possibilities of change. In June 2000, the Department of Health and Human Services, with the leadership of Secretary Donna Shalala, began to remodel the nation's human research system under the director of its new Office for Human Research Protection. Progress has been rapid. Just two years later, Senator Bill Frist of Tennessee, who had chaired an earlier series of hearings that sparked the reform effort, listened to witnesses from the pharmaceutical industry, the academic community, and from advocacy groups. "We are not where we were," he remarked, but added that there was still a long way to go.[5]

The Myth of Compliance

What are the precepts on which reform should be based? Again, it helps to review fundamental principles. Laws and regulations are created when people won't do things they should do and are too willing to do things they should not do. Notice the emphasis on "should." There is an ethical implication based on a concept of right behavior and wrong behavior. In effect, we are trying to promote responsible, ethical conduct. Unfortunately, when we live within a legal framework, we don't necessarily end up with responsible, ethical conduct; instead, we often wind up with noncompliance with regulations. Researchers may not be aware of or understand the regulations. They may lack the necessary training or resources to comply. Some may lack the commitment. Faced with an array of detailed, bewildering regulations, many human beings are inclined to disregard them and simply do as they please. But the problem runs deeper than this.

Even if we had full compliance with laws and regulations, there is no reason to believe that human subjects would be fully protected. Think of an analogous situation. The Joint Committee on Accreditation of Healthcare Organizations visits a hospital for an audit. The auditors check to see that there are no beds in the hallway. They check to see that equipment works properly. They check to see that the hospital has an ethics committee. But even if the hospital passes all these tests with flying colors, there is no guarantee that it is capable of delivering high-quality medical care. So it is with scientific research. Even if a researcher has every consent form properly signed and dated, there is no guarantee that a truly effective process of informed consent was conducted. Even if an IRB has signed off on every research protocol, there is no guarantee that the research will actually be conducted ethically and safely. The myth of compliance is that compliance will achieve the results we desire. Unfortunately, it is just that, a myth.

Laws and regulations may actually make things worse. After all, the implementation of laws and regulations requires resources. An organization cannot establish an IRB without giving it the resources it needs to function. But if the laws and regulations are poorly designed in the first place, those resources are being spent on the wrong thing. Moreover, the compliance process seems to have a built-in logic that requires more and more regulations and more and more resources. In the past few years, institutions have scrambled to make their programs compliant, beefing up their review boards and erecting more and more requirements for would-be researchers. In doing so, they have created greater impediments to conducting research in a responsible manner, but there is no evidence to show that improved compliance translates to a more effective system. If more laws and regulations are not the answer, what is?

Culture of Conscience

The desired outcome of the human-research endeavor is clear: to facilitate the conduct of responsible research in such a way that no one is ever harmed, if possible. Prevention of harm—true protection of human subjects—is a critical element of an effective and trustworthy research system, as is efficiency in the research process. To reach this outcome, I would argue that we must take a giant step backward to where the scientific community was in 1966 and take a different path. The new path would lead not to a culture of compliance, which is a failed model, but to a *culture of conscience*.[6]

In a culture of conscience, people act responsibly because it is the right thing to do, rather than because the government tells them to do so. Responsibility includes inviting scrutiny. Because researchers are making every effort to do things right, they invite people to look at what they are doing. A culture of conscience also means that people are accountable for what they do. As Ronald Reagan said of his approach to the Soviet Union over disarmament, "Trust, but verify." Accountability, or verification, is the counterpart of responsibility. Both demand openness and honesty in the entire process.

The public—people outside the research community, including patients and their families—is necessarily a partner in this process. This is a big change, and a controversial one. In the past, the public was simply a source of research subjects. Today, lay people want a voice in what research will be conducted and in how it will be conducted. Public involvement is controversial because many scientists believe that nonprofessionals cannot understand all the complexities involved and so will be just one more barrier. If the public does not understand research, how can it learn to trust the researchers? If the public does not trust the researchers, it will make certain that the barriers to research are very high.

Some kind of partnership with the public is inevitable, whatever researchers may think of it, and there are reasons to believe that the effects will be positive. Consider the tragic event some years ago at the Dana Farber Cancer Institute in Boston. A health and science reporter for the *Boston Globe,* Betsy Lehman, was being treated for cancer and was given, in error, an incorrect dose of medicine. She died as a result of the error. It was a classic case of a poor system leading to an adverse outcome. But because of that tragic event, Dana Farber invited members of the patient community and their families to sit on a board that would scrutinize adverse events and help determine how to improve the systems that led to them. That single step has probably done more to revitalize the institution, to build the faith and trust of its patient community, than any other step Dana Farber could have taken.

A New Paradigm

In the aftermath of tragedy, a new paradigm has begun to emerge. The old paradigm was protectionism through laws and regulations. The investigators, the sponsors, and the research team were trying to conduct the research. The IRBs were attempting to provide oversight and accountability. The public, including patients, their families, and the media, was on the outside looking in. It was fundamentally a confrontational model, with the researchers separated from subjects by the familiar twin pillars, or twin barriers. It was also a model based on mistrust. The new paradigm recognizes that every party to the research process shares a primary responsibility for protecting the interests and well-being of the research participants and for ensuring that research is done efficiently as well as ethically. That changes the entire spectrum of relationships because it establishes shared *goals*. No longer is the IRB the sole body with primary responsibility for the protection of human subjects. That is now the job of everybody involved in the research, as is timely performance.

Implementation of the new paradigm involves a number of different elements, together composing a *program*, with individual programs linked as components of a *system*. Review boards in one form or another will not disappear. In human research, there will always be a need for some element of peer review, just because we humans are imperfect and will always need oversight. But the review board may need to be more independent of the sponsoring institution so that it can focus on reviewing the research without potential conflicts of interest or commitment. The reviewers will need extensive specialized training in both ethics and science to do their jobs, as practiced in other safety-critical industries, such as aviation. Greater reliance on expert consultation will facilitate the review process and improve its effectiveness. The review boards will also need resources, staffing, information systems, and communications systems. They cannot function effectively without this kind of organizational support and without the resources required to maintain the support.

In each program, other activities will interface with the review process. For example, organizations may conduct compliance oversight or quality assurance processes to ensure that ongoing research is conducted properly, not just approved and forgotten. Adverse events must be monitored and acted on as they occur. Treated properly, adverse event reporting can feed in to quality review and so ultimately lead to performance improvements. The inevitable potential for conflicts of interest means that there must be a process for disclosure and for management of potential conflicts. That should not be the sole responsibility of the research review board. Finally, the process requires education at a variety of levels. People need to learn and to understand what they are expected to do so that they can actually do it. The goal, again, should not be cast as a negative one, that is, protecting human subjects from research. Rather, the goal should be to promote responsible research, recognizing that responsible research strives to prevent harm to human subjects. Most people have good intentions. If they are committed to a known goal and if they are given the resources, they will accomplish it.

Performance and Compliance

This paradigm can be divided into two domains, a performance domain and a compliance domain. Ideally, we want to focus on the performance domain—to develop systems that align incentives and encourage behavior focused on excellence and trust. Right now we are beginning to see the development of independent, private, voluntary accreditation and certification programs. Such programs afford opportunities for the research community to demonstrate its commitment to excellence voluntarily, without coercion of the law. These tools have been used effectively in industry, in education, and in many professions. Such efforts are validation activities. They say, in effect, that the organization is doing things right. Obtaining such validation provides a positive incentive for organizations and researchers, not just the negative incentive of having to meet regulatory requirements. Such programs also foster trust. Consultation between the government and the private sector as these programs develop can help ensure that they are used effectively and without duplication.

If efforts to adopt performance standards fail; if the research community fails to implement them; or if we cannot measure their impact, then we will likely return to the compliance domain. Compliance oversight includes investigation, which is one thing that regulatory agencies do on a daily basis, when responding to an adverse event or complaint. It also includes what might be called not-for-cause evaluations, which in the business world is known as quality control. That means proactively evaluating ongoing research projects and procedures in order to identify problems and develop systems to improve them *before* something bad happens. The balance between performance efforts and compliance efforts will depend very much on how many episodes of irresponsible behavior come to light. The more episodes there are, the more we will have to rely on compliance and enforcement activities.

More Challenges and Opportunities

Despite the emergence of this new paradigm, our system for human research continues to face a variety of challenges and opportunities.

The Janus Phenomenon

Janus, the god of gates and doorways, was a Greek mythological figure with two faces, each looking in the opposite direction. Government agencies often find themselves in much the same position. The Department of Health and Human Services (HHS), the world's largest research funding agency and home to the National Institutes of Health (NIH), the world's largest research facility, is also charged with oversight of that research. For nearly 30 years, the Office for Protection from Research Risks, OHRP's predecessor, was located in NIH, which meant that the oversight agency was actually reporting to the director of the funding agency. Any agency with competing goals may find it difficult to pursue both effectively; HHS is not alone in its predicament.

The Federal "Anti-Commons"

Science is conducted with a notion of an "intellectual commons," a collaborative pursuit of knowledge and truth based on sharing information. This has been the basis for scientific progress over the years. Government rarely works on this basis, as we have seen in our pursuit of homeland security, statutes, regulations, and administrative complexity. All erect barriers to cooperation and the open sharing of information, even when it is desirable and appropriate. Similar problems occur in any large bureaucratic organization, such as a university or a hospital. Developing systems that work together for the common good in this context can be difficult, but the benefit is likely to be worth the effort.

The "Uncommon Paradox" of the Common Rule

The regulations for protection of human subjects were originally promulgated by what was then the Department of Health, Education and Welfare, now HHS. After a 10-year effort, 17 federal agencies agreed to adopt the HHS rules, creating what has become known as the common rule, to provide an integrated approach, even though each agency is permitted to interpret the rules differently. Paradoxically, the common rule has become an impediment to integration because any changes to the policy require clearance and approval from 17 agencies (some of them with heads looking in opposite directions!). Consequently, some have called for adoption of a single policy by statute, and a single, independent oversight agency. Such legislation has already been introduced in Congress.

The Big Brother Effect

When systems begin to fail, the Big Brother effect kicks in. If the regulations already in place are not sufficient to get the job done, let's have more regulations or even fines and other penalties for noncompliance. Fearful of enforcement activities, institutions and IRBs have resorted to a state of reactive hyperprotectionism. Faced with this phenomenon, many research scientists find that the barriers are higher and higher and that the research is harder and harder to do. If the government follows the same course, there is likely to be a far-reaching negative impact on human research for generations to come. And going back is not easy.

Earning Trust

The consequences of failing to restore and rebuild trust in human research may be profound. In a worst-case scenario, we can imagine that a clinical trial is announced and no one—no one—volunteers. People would say, "I'm sorry, I don't trust this process, and I am not going to take part." The impact of that on the progress of biomedical research and biomedical science would be devastating. Many have feared, in the recent past, that that is exactly where we were heading. Our hope with the new paradigm is to turn it around and to move in the right direction. If it works, what one can imagine is more positive.[7] Imagine, for instance, that physician investigators were true academicians, driven not by the funds brought in for enrolling patients in a clinical trial but by the pure quest for knowledge to improve care. Imagine that physicians who wanted to start a company and hold equity in it took leaves of absence from the academic community to avoid any possibility of conflicting interests. Imagine that the process of reviewing human research and protecting human subjects was recognized and appreciated in the academic culture for what it is, an intrinsic part of the research process. Building trust in research may actually encourage more people to participate.

On the industry side, imagine that a pharmaceutical company designs a protocol not simply to get the data necessary for drug approval, but first for the well-being of potential subjects. In fact, we may not be so far away from such a shift. In our post-Enron world, more and more companies are beginning to recognize that there is a business value in protecting the trust consumers put in them. Pharmaceutical and medical-device companies are beginning to acknowledge that properly done research is more valuable than haphazard or unethical research and that doing things right actually enhances their value as businesses. Already, pharmaceutical companies have adopted a new code of ethics for conducting clinical trials and new guidelines for interaction among sales representatives and physicians. How effective these changes will be remains to be seen. Meanwhile, groups such as the American Academy of Pharmaceutical Physicians and the Association of Clinical Research Professionals are developing more rigorous standards, creating programs for training and certification of individuals doing research, and endorsing private accreditation of research programs.

Trust, like respect, is not something that anybody can demand. Nor is it something that can be imposed through regulations and laws. Trust must be earned. The shift from focusing on noncompliance to focusing on excellence and responsibility is critically important to establishing trust. Accountability, validation, and the openness that both require are the tools with which trust can be built.

Notes

1. Michael De. Lemonick and Andrew Goldstein, "At Your Own Risk," *Time,* April 22, 2002.

2. Henry K Beecher, "Ethics in Clinical Research," *New England Journal of Medicine* 278 (1966): 1425–1430.

3. Eric G. Campbell, Gred Koski, Darren E. Zinner, and David Blumenthal, "Managing the Triple Helix in the Life Sciences," *Issues in Science and Technology* 21 (2005): 48–54.

4. June Gibbs Brown, "Institutional Review Boards: A Time for Reform," Department of Health and Human Services, June 1998. Publication #OEI-01–97–00193. Available: http://oig.hhs.gov/oei/reports/oei-01–97–00193.pdf (accessed April 21, 2006).

5. I relate Senator Frist's comment in my resignation letter to Secretary Tommy Thompson, when I stepped down as the first director of the Office for Human Research Protections in 2002. Available: http://irb.mc.duke.edu/PDF/koskiLetter.pdf (accessed April 21, 2006).

6. A return to the same "culture of conscience" of the mid-1960s would be difficult. In the intervening decades, the growing industry-university ties have imbued research with a profit motive and various conflicts of interest. However, a new type of conscience can be developed in lieu of regulation. See Greg Koski, "Research, Regulations, and Responsibility: Confronting the Compliance Myth—A Reaction to Professor Gatter," *Emory Law Journal* 52 (2003): 403–416.

7. Greg Koski, "Imagination and Attention: Protecting Participants in Psychopharmacological Research," *Psychopharmacology* 171 (2003): 56–57.

9

Medical Education: Teaching Doctors to Be Trustworthy

JORDAN J. COHEN

Why must patients trust their doctors? Surely one answer is that there is a deep psychological need for trust in times of vulnerability, such as during an illness or after an injury. It is a trait that probably hearkens back to prehistory, when we placed our trust in the shamans. When we are sick, we want to believe that someone can and will take care of us. Then, too, trust is a prerequisite for effective care. Patients must reveal to their doctors aspects of their personal health that are usually kept private and so must trust that physicians will treat their information with respect and confidentiality. Patients also must comply with what their physicians or other caregivers recommend for their care. That often entails a measure of risk, and patients must trust that the risk is appropriate and considered. Moreover, patients' and doctors' ability to form trusting, caring relationships itself has therapeutic benefits and can have a positive effect on medical outcomes.

But there is another way of looking at the benefits of trust. Consider the problem of safeguarding patients' welfare when they enter this complex, risky, error-prone enterprise known as modern healthcare. We can pass laws and regulations spelling out what caregivers can and cannot do. We can establish a patients' bill of rights, spelling out patients' entitlements. We can establish watchdog federal agencies, such as the Food and Drug Administration and the Office of the Inspector General, and we can fill insurance policies with fine print that details what will and will not be covered. While all these measures have a role to play, they are blunt and often ineffective instruments. The legal system, for example, may be able to help patients recover damages after the fact, but it cannot effectively protect them in the course of care. Watchdog agencies can focus on finding the bad apples or cheats, and they can help to maintain compliance with regulations, but again they cannot greatly affect what happens to an individual patient in an encounter with the system. Nor can the insurance companies, which in fact usually try to avoid taking responsibility when bad things happen during individual encounters.

The fact is that none of these tools, however useful, comes close to being as effective a safeguard as trust in one's doctor. Physicians' trustworthiness provides the most effective, durable, and reliable safeguard against the inherent dangers in modern therapeutics. Without trust, we are all in trouble.

To date, the data suggest that patients still have a great deal of confidence in their own physicians. In one survey using a five-point scale, with five indicating complete agreement, the statement "My doctor really cares about me as a person" scores 4.4. The statement "My doctor puts my needs first" scores 4.1, and "My doctor keeps my information totally private" scores 4.4.[1] These high scores are hardly surprising, given the need to trust a physician when one is sick. But trust in the healthcare system as a whole, as has been noted elsewhere in this book, has been declining for decades. Today, only about 30 percent of the public expresses a great deal of confidence in medicine. That is surely a cause for alarm.

The Role of Medical Education

It is not immediately obvious what medical education can do to address this problem. A skeptical view would suggest that no one can be taught to be trustworthy, certainly not at the relatively advanced age of the average medical student. Trustworthiness, in this view, is taught in the sandbox and at the family dinner table or not at all. Indeed, there are some 25-year-olds whom no one could teach to be trustworthy. They simply do not have the necessary character and integrity. But people who enter medicine with the right attitudes, motivations, and values—most medical students, in other words—seem to me quite different. Anyone who has spent a career in medical education knows that appropriate approaches can indeed nurture and sustain trustworthiness in these people.

Appropriate Admissions Criteria

By and large, acceptance into medical school is tantamount to acceptance into the medical profession. Very few people wash out; only four to five percent of students accepted to medical school do not earn an M.D. degree, and most of those who leave do so for financial or personal reasons, such as deciding that they did not want to be doctors. Admissions committees understand this and in general do a reasonable job of assessing not just academic credentials but character traits that affect trustworthiness and the ability to establish caring relationships. Since the applicant pool is still roughly twice as large as the number of available positions, admissions committees do make choices. And because the applicant pool is self-selected, the committees are generally choosing among highly gifted and motivated individuals.

Nevertheless, I believe we could do an even better job. Medical schools in general tend to convey the message to pre-med students that they are not as interested in applicants' character as they are in their academic performance, for example, in fields such as organic chemistry. Admissions committees could do a much better job of signaling to undergraduates that they are looking for intelligent idealists, not simply bright students capable of achieving a 4.0 grade point average. Schools do want people with the compassion, the leadership qualities, and the understanding of the doctor-patient relationship that will allow them to become trustworthy physicians. Medical schools should let applicants know that.[2]

Explicit Learning Objectives

The theory of adult learning is unambiguous: if people are presented with prospective learning objectives, if they understand what the faculty and the institution expect of them during the course of their education, it is far more likely that they will achieve those objectives. Because they know what is expected of them, they find ways to accomplish those objectives. The formal curriculum has an important role to play here. The cognitive rationale for trust in the doctor-patient relationship must be established, and historical references and case studies can help provide it. But the informal curriculum may be even more important. People learn the norms of their profession by observing how their professors and other physicians conduct themselves.[3]

It is in the informal curriculum that schools face the biggest challenge: they must ensure that the learning environments to which students are exposed are suffused with the ethical and professional norms that inculcate trustworthiness. Their ability to do this has suffered in recent years, as market forces have begun to change medicine dramatically. It is hard to maintain the traditional professional paradigm when there is so much emphasis in the external world on the commercial paradigm.

Evaluation and Reward of Behaviors and Attitudes

A medical school's tools for evaluating, say, a student's ability to do a lumbar puncture are usually quite good. Even communication skills can be assessed relatively easily. Evaluating traits such as trustworthiness is much harder. The keys would seem to be identifying desirable behaviors when they are seen, rewarding them appropriately, and sanctioning behaviors that are not consistent with professional norms. That combination of reward and sanction can help students understand that how they act is as important as the procedures they learn to perform. Too often in learning environments, faculty members countenance incompetence, surliness, and other inappropriate behavior. The offender may be a friend and colleague. It may be awkward to confront them. Still, every interaction is a lesson that a student is learning. It is important that those lessons be the ones we strive to teach.

Articulation of Explicit Institutional Expectations: The Model Compact

The leadership of a medical school—indeed, the leadership of any institution—should go on record with what the institution stands for and what it expects.

A good example of this approach is the model Compact Between Teachers and Learners of Medicine, prepared by the Association of American Medical Colleges (AAMC) and distributed at the association's annual meeting in 2001. The preamble to the compact states the matter squarely: "Preparation for a career in medicine demands the acquisition of a large fund of knowledge and a host of special skills. It also demands the strengthening of those virtues that undergird the doctor/patient relationship and that sustain the profession of medicine as a moral enterprise. This Compact serves both as a pledge and as a reminder to teachers and learners that their conduct in fulfilling their mutual obligations is the medium through which the profession inculcates its ethical values."[4]

The compact then goes on to cite three guiding principles that underline the issues. One is *duty:* Medical educators have a duty to their students not only to convey the knowledge and skills required of a doctor but also to teach those values and attitudes that are required to preserve medicine's social contract. The second is *integrity,* or a consistency between what one says and what one does: "Students learn enduring lessons of professionalism by observing and emulating role models who epitomize authentic professional values and attitudes." The third is *respect.* In the hierarchy between teachers and learners there is a gradient of authority, and that gradient gives rise to the possibility of exploitation, abuse, and arrogance. But mutual respect is critical to learning, and teachers have a special obligation to treat students and residents respectfully.

The compact also includes a series of commitments. Faculty are asked to pledge that they will in fact offer a high standard of instruction; that they will maintain high professional standards in their interactions with patients, colleagues, and staff; that they will respect students and residents as individuals, without regard to gender, race, or other social variables; and that they will not tolerate the manifestation of disrespect or bias by others. Faculty members also pledge that students and residents will have sufficient time to fulfill personal and family obligations. This last pledge is critically important in an environment that for many years has been characterized by excessive hours and demands. Moderating those demands is conducive to patient safety, and it helps promote the health and well-being of the caregivers.

Finally, the faculty pledges to celebrate "expressions of professional attitudes and behaviors" as well as academic achievement, and it pledges not to tolerate abuse or exploitation of students or residents: "We encourage any student or resident who experiences mistreatment or who witnesses unprofessional behavior to report the facts immediately to appropriate faculty or staff . . . [W]e treat all such reports as confidential and do not tolerate reprisals or retaliations of any kind." As with the new approach toward errors in medical care, the attempt here is to make certain that problems can be addressed without fear of retribution.

Students and residents are asked to make a similar set of commitments. They pledge that they will work hard to acquire the knowledge, skills, attitudes, and behaviors established by the faculty. They pledge to "cherish the professional virtues of honesty, compassion, integrity, fidelity, and dependability." They pledge respect to all, and they pledge to conduct themselves in accordance with the "highest standards of the medical profession in all their interactions." They also pledge that they will assist their fellow students and residents in meeting their professional obligations.

Next Steps

It is not yet clear how many medical schools have adopted this compact, though some have at least circulated and discussed it. At any rate, its importance lies not in the details but in the principle, namely that an institution needs to articulate in very clear terms its expectations of its faculty, residents, and students. Such a step will help ratify an individual's own inclinations to do the right thing. Most people would like to act within the norms of the profession. A compact such as this does not provide a roadmap or a template for behavior, but it does legitimize people's wishes to act in desirable ways.

Also to this end, the AAMC has recently launched the Institute for the Improvement of Medical Education. Medical education is often perceived by the public as an archaic institution mired in the Flexner Report era. Certainly, many medical schools have been less than nimble in responding to the astonishing changes that have taken place in healthcare over the past hundred years. But there is more change taking place in medical education than may be apparent, and much of it is driven by the recognition that professionalism and trustworthiness do not necessarily rank as highly as they should. The compact and the new institute are both attempts to address that failing. So too are a series of national awards sponsored by the AAMC, including annual humanism awards for individual students and community service awards for institutions.

One additional initiative deserves mention: in conjunction with the American Board of Internal Medicine Foundation, the AAMC is developing measures of professionalism that can be used to assess progress toward the competencies described in this chapter.[5] A useful tool in this arena may be peer evaluation. Already we expect professionals throughout their careers to evaluate one another for board certification, licensure, hospital privileges, and so on. But we have neglected the opportunity to introduce peer evaluations to help people learn and monitor the traits of professionalism and trustworthiness. Such peer review can articulate these important values and operationalize the expectations of the profession.

Ultimately, of course, trust is earned, not owed. Many in medicine have been lulled into the belief that trust is owed just because healthcare is so important to people. But that is a dangerous attitude; it creates a sense of complacency and a sense of entitlement. The public no longer accepts the idea that it owes trust to physicians and other caregivers. Of course, earning trust is difficult. All the initiatives and compacts and principles in the world will not suffice if individual students and individual physicians do not learn to act in a trustworthy manner. But I believe that trustworthiness can be learned, and that trust can be earned by being trustworthy.

In closing, I offer a few practical suggestions to medical-school faculty and others on how to be a positive influence on medical students:

- In case discussions, identify instances in which lack of trust between patient and physician resulted in substandard care.
- Create a simulated patient case for educational purposes in which students are expected to establish a trusting relationship with a mistrustful patient.
- In medical humanities courses, select illustrative literature for discussion of the importance of trust between doctor and patient and between the medical profession and society.
- In personal dealings with patients, model the professional attributes that sustain trust— for example, protection of patient privacy; consideration for patients' time when scheduling appointments; respect for patients' autonomy in decisions about their care; honesty in the face of medical error; and sensitivity to cultural differences.

Notes

1. Adapted from David H. Thom et al., "Further Validation and Reliability of the Trust in Physician Scale," *Medical Care* (1999) 37: 510–517.

2. Jill Gordon, "Fostering Students' Personal and Professional Development in Medicine: A New Framework for PPD," *Medical Education* 37 (2003): 341–349.

3. N. P. Kenny, K. V. Mann et al., "Role Modeling in Physicians' Professional Formation," *Academic Medicine* 78 (2003): 1203–1210.

4. Association of American Medical Colleges, "Compact between Teachers and Learners of Medicine." Available: http://www.aamc.org/newsroom/pressrel/compact.pdf (accessed April 19, 2006).

5. L. S. Robbins, C. H. Braddock III et al., "Using the American Board of Internal Medicine's 'Elements of Professional' for Undergraduate Ethics Education," *Academic Medicine* 77 (2002): 523–531.

10

Trustworthy Information:
Medical Journals and the Internet

GEORGE D. LUNDBERG

In his initial address to the membership of the Institute of Medicine in 2002, incoming president Harvey Fineberg described what he called a medical perfect storm. The number of uninsured in the United States had risen sharply. The cost of healthcare was again spiraling out of control. There were profound questions about the quality of care, indeed about basic patient safety. As if this triangulation of trouble were not enough, Dr. Fineberg could easily have expanded the list of concerns. The pharmaceutical industry is today under unprecedented public and political attack. Approval ratings for the for-profit managed care industry are about on par with those of tobacco companies. The cost of professional liability coverage has some medical specialties in a stranglehold. Many academic medical centers are in precarious financial condition. Aware of these troubles, the best and brightest college graduates in recent years have begun voting with their feet; they are applying to law schools and business schools instead of to medical schools.

And yet individual physicians have somehow, miraculously, maintained a relationship with the public characterized by high levels of trust. Though trust levels have decreased for many groups, including hospitals and health insurance companies, doctors still rank high in the public's estimation. Whether physicians can continue to merit this level of trust, of course, is uncertain. The answer may depend largely on whether they can lead the public out of the morass that healthcare has become and help create a new and better system. My colleagues and I have offered proposals for a new system in the paperback version of my book *Severed Trust: Why American Medicine Hasn't Been Fixed*. In this chapter, I limn the outlines of this system by focusing on a central feature of any workable system: trustworthy information.[1]

Trust in the Published Word

It is said that we are in the midst of an information revolution, and indeed we are. But the roots of this revolution do not extend back only to the invention of the Internet; they go back to the invention of the movable-type printing press. The first explosive growth of information coincided with the ability to disseminate that information easily and cheaply to a wide readership through the printed word. The development of the printing press coincided with the widespread adoption of the scientific method, in which experimental results were published for all to see and to attempt to replicate. The chief vehicle for the dissemination of scientific information became the peer-reviewed journal.

Peer review, invented almost simultaneously in England and France some 300 years ago, is a simple enough procedure. A journal editor submits manuscripts to acknowledged experts inside or outside the editorial office for their considered opinions and recommendations on publication. Yet peer review is one of many social inventions whose simplicity belies their importance. Scientific experimenters hope to achieve a given result through a given method. But since scientists are human beings, they are prone to wishful thinking, sloppy hypotheses, methodological errors, and many other research sins. Peer review holds their work to a high standard. If the authors of a scientific paper posit a linkage of cause and effect, they cannot simply observe that event B happened after event A. They must also explain why A caused B, they must rule out alternative causes of B, and they must do whatever else may be necessary to produce a valid conclusion. This is particularly important for the experimental scientists known as physicians, who do many things to patients, hoping to achieve certain results, and who often overestimate or misinterpret the effects of their actions. (Samuel Johnson said, "It is incident to physicians I am afraid beyond all other men to mistake subsequence for consequence."[2]) Peer review endeavors to ensure that claims about the effectiveness or ineffectiveness of medical procedures are substantiated, that they can be trusted.

The editor of a peer-reviewed medical journal relies on experts to assess the trustworthiness of a paper: Are the data accurate? Are the conclusions justified by the data? The editor also depends upon these experts to answer many other questions: Is the material original? Is it important? Is it interesting, clearly presented, and timely? As one editor put it, it is the job of experts to gauge whether a contribution is both new and true. *True,* of course, means true for the moment. No editor, indeed no panel of experts, can certify that a paper's findings will be true forever; another paper may be published tomorrow that utilizes different research methodologies and finds different answers. But the peer review process attests, in effect, that the authors have adhered to the standards of the scientific method and that their conclusions are our best approximation of the truth at this time.

Peer review is a necessary but insufficient condition for a medical journal's trustworthiness. For example, what happens when something goes wrong in the publishing process? Perhaps a name is printed incorrectly. Perhaps an X-ray is published backwards. If a paper is marred by an honest error, reputable journals publish corrections as quickly as possible. If a paper is found to be fraudulent, reputable journals retract it entirely. (They do not publish corrections if new information comes out the next day, simply because the literature is expected to correct itself in this manner.) Moreover, no journal is simply a link between authors, reviewers, and readers. When I was editor of *The Journal of the American Medical Association* (JAMA), I felt that I was at the center of a "wheel of trust," involving not just these groups but also institutions, funding agencies, students, advertisers, sponsors, and the organization that owned the journal. In a sense, it is the editor's job to maintain trust among all these groups, even though many of them are likely to be in disagreement much of the time.

The editor of a medical journal has one more significant relationship of trust, namely the relationship between the information he or she is responsible for publishing and the patients who may be affected by it. This is a curious relationship, because, at least until the advent of the electronic age, patients would rarely see the information. Still, every editor must ask whether the article they are considering publishing will beneficial to patients in some way or potentially harmful., That is the ultimate basis for every decision.

The Medical Internet

In recent years, the rather staid world of medical journals has been supplanted or at least supplemented by the Internet as a primary source of medical information. And what a source it is. The Internet consists of a web of networks, millions and millions of participants, uncounted research databases, numberless articles, and floods of snippets, tips, and factoids. It is voluminous, interactive, worldwide, and searchable—a truly massive information source, surely the most important development in human communication since the printing press. About one-third of Americans access the Internet regularly; that number will surely rise over time. Of course, the Internet is also unregulated, and much of the information on it is untrustworthy.[3] But to criticize it on these grounds is to mistake the medium for the message. Printed information is unregulated as well, and much of it is untrustworthy.[4] To say I don't believe anything I read on the Internet makes as much sense as saying I don't believe anything I read on paper. The real question is, "How can interested people find trustworthy information on the Internet?"[5] In other words, what is the functional equivalent of peer review?

Because the Internet is so new, it may help to step back and look at how trustworthiness in general is established. Aside from our genetic makeup and our early learning, there are three essential controllers of human behavior. One is personal morality—our ideas about right human conduct, about what it is to be good. If personal morality were strong enough, there would be no need for anything else. But because we human beings are fallible, we rely on two other methods of control, ethics and law. Ethics are principles of conduct that govern groups of people.

Laws are rules that are formally recognized as binding and that are backed up by the force of central authority. People trust one another, when they agree that one or more of these forces will govern their behavior. In the case of medical journals, we assume the information is trustworthy primarily because it is governed by a code of ethics that has evolved over centuries and that most people involved in journals take very seriously.

Some years back—a century in Internet time, but in reality only a few years— several groups of people who were involved in the medical Internet sat down to write a code of ethics that we hoped would govern it. We began with the same concept that underlies peer review, namely, that the essence of professionalism is self-governance. Nobody wanted laws and regulations governing the medical Internet; we wanted it to be governed by professionals. Given that starting point, there was much we could draw from other fields.

The Medical Internet Is Medicine

The American Medical Association was founded in 1846, and one of its objectives was to develop a code of ethics for the American medical profession. And it did. The most up-to-date and comprehensive statement of these ethics is contained in the *Code of Medical Ethics: Current Opinions,* from the AMA's Council on Ethical and Judicial Affairs. By now, this is a book of more than 200 pages, but it boils down to doing the right thing for individual patients and populations of patients. This was a principle that we believed should inform the ethics of the medical Internet.

The Medical Internet Is Journalism

The Society of Professional Journalists issued a code of ethics in 1996 that includes 77 points under the following four categories: Seek truth and report it; minimize harm; act independently; and hold yourself accountable. These, too, were principles we believed should inform the medical Internet's ethics.

The Medical Internet Is Business

Those who have lost a lot of money on medical Web sites may take issue with this statement. But business it is, and indeed it has been a good business for some companies. Business, too, has its ethics. In 1924, for example, the U.S. Chamber of Commerce issued 15 principles of business conduct. It banned actions such as bribery and fraud. But it also included statements such as this: "It is a moral obligation of individuals who work in the business to do the right thing, even if the business does the wrong thing." In other words, it legitimized whistle-blowing. It also stated, "Business should render restrictive legislation unnecessary." In other words, the observance of a code of ethics should be sufficient to regulate behavior.

The Medical Internet Is Medical Journalism

The rules for medical journalism are written by the International Committee of Medical Journal Editors (ICMJE), known as the Vancouver Group, which consists of editors of the main general medical journals from around the world. The group was founded in 1978—300 years after the beginning of peer review!—and meets roughly once a year to update the rules.

The Medical Internet Is Medical Education

We drew on a document called the Ethics of Medical Education from the Accreditation Council for Continuing Medical Education (ACCME). My own company, Medscape (owned at this writing by WebMD), offers many different kinds of continuing medical education courses, and is utilized for this purpose by medical professionals all over the country. ACCME rules inform our operation and the operation of many other continuing-education companies.

Out of the effort to develop ethics for the medical Internet came five different codes. The office of Senator Joseph Lieberman of Connecticut rolled out a code on Capitol Hill in May 2000. It included eight domains: candor, honesty, quality, informed consent, privacy, professionalism, responsible partnering, and accountability. The same month, in San Francisco, a group known as High Ethics produced a 14-point policy on how the medical Internet should be governed. Other groups have also created codes of ethical conduct, including the ICMJE itself, the AMA, and the American Accreditation Healthcare Commission, known as URAC.

Will it work? A few years ago, we at Medscape published a survey on our Web site asking our 4.5 million registrants in 237 countries how they would judge the ethics of a medical Web site. Thousands responded. Only 9 percent said they would rely on brand-name identification, and only 15 percent said they would rely on an ethics statement or seal of approval. A much larger group, 44 percent, responded that they would rely on implied endorsement by leading experts. (The rest had no opinion or said they didn't know.) We repeated the identical survey in late 2002. The results were virtually unchanged. We hope that many sites and organizations adopt and practice an appropriate code of ethics to assure users that their information is trustworthy.

E-Care: System of the Future?

I have focused on the medical Internet because I believe that it is likely to be at the core of the evolving healthcare system in the United States, and so the trustworthiness of the information provided and exchanged over the Internet is a critical issue. In theory, the Internet allows us to have 280 million individual health plans, one for every man, woman, and child in the United States. Exactly what such a system would look like, of course, remains to be seen. But I believe it is possible to christen the system (I call it "e-care") and to outline its central principles.

Universal Health Insurance by Individual Mandate

Under e-care, everyone is required to have health insurance. No country in the world has ever achieved universal coverage except by a mandate, and in the United States the individual mandate must be established and enforced by federal law. The concept is much the same as mandatory licensing and insurance for drivers: Just as you cannot operate a car without a driver's license and auto insurance, so you cannot be a resident of the nation without health insurance. The actual provision of insurance could come in many forms. Employer-based insurance is one mechanism for providing it. Medicaid and Medicare are others. People could buy insurance for themselves.

Cost Control through Market Forces

There are only two ways to control costs in healthcare. The government can take it over and set all the rates, as is the case in some countries. Most Americans do not favor such a system, so it seems wise to search for an alternative. The only effective alternative I know of is to rely on market forces. Insurance policies would therefore carry a high deductible, perhaps between $1,000 and $3,000 a year in 2006 dollars, with supplements from the government for low-income families. With such a deductible, most ambulatory care would be paid out of the patient's own pocket, which means that patients would have to become wiser consumers of healthcare. Our current system could be called "uninformed consent"; few people really know or care how much a given procedure or visit will cost, because insurance pays all or nearly all the cost. In e-care, the doctor or other caregiver informs nonemergency patients what a procedure is going to cost, and the patient decides whether he or she wants it. We call this economic informed consent.

Protection against Catastrophe

In e-care, hospital or other catastrophic care above the yearly deductible is paid entirely by insurance. There are no more co-pays and there is no additional deductible. Nor is there a lifetime cap. Granted, all such mechanisms help to control costs. But they also expose patients to unacceptable financial risk. No American should have to become bankrupt because of medical expenses.

Preventive Medicine Is Public Health

The claim is made that, if people are buying their own medical care, nobody will be willing to pay for preventive measures. But scientifically proven prevention should be called public health, and the government should pay for it because it is in the country's best interest. No one argues against using the government's funds to ensure clean water or sewage disposal; by the same token, it is in our national interest to do what we can to reduce the toll taken by heart disease, cancer, and stroke. When preventive interventions against such killers are supported by solid scientific evidence, the preventive actions should be sponsored and paid for by the government.

Quality and Safety Concerns

The Institute of Medicine issued three landmark reports, in 1999, 2001, and 2002 on error prevention and quality assurance. The recommendations in those reports need to be implemented and enforced. This will require a commitment and a level of funding from Congress that goes well beyond what is currently available. To offer just one recommendation, the Food and Drug Administration should require testing of proposed drug names to eliminate names that sound or look alike, thereby helping to avoid confusion in the writing and filling of prescriptions.

Privacy and Confidentiality

As more and more information is exchanged over the Internet, people are rightly concerned about privacy and confidentiality. Of course, these concerns did not originate with electronic communication; they have been around as long as there have been hospitals, perhaps as long as there have been physicians. Right now, large quantities of information about patients are captured and contained in databases maintained by doctors' offices, hospitals, insurance companies, and pharmaceutical companies. People who truly want information to be kept private are obliged to pay their doctor in cash and ask that the record be kept out of the main database.

The Internet does not change this situation much. Firewalls and other security devices can help protect electronic information from random snooping. Ethics codes and the new confidentiality rules established by the Health Insurance Portability and Accountability Act (HIPAA) can discourage it. Even so, there is no guarantee—just as there is no guarantee now—that all information will be totally private and confidential.

The Future

I have a vision of a new world made better largely by information. To be sure, it is a vision that smacks of utopianism in a world where 50 percent of the population suffers from malnourishment, 80 percent live in substandard housing, 70 percent are unable to read, and only 1 percent has a college education or owns a computer. But progress depends on grand visions, and we live at a time when the opportunities for change have expanded as never before. E-care is a system in which information is offered and exchanged with remarkable ease. All the more important, therefore, that the information be trustworthy.

Action Items for Clinicians to Establish Trust

- Work actively to establish universal access to basic care for all Americans.
- Except in emergencies, disclose and discuss costs of medical care before administering it.
- Be competent and ethical in your practices, including practicing evidence-based medicine.
- Recognize that most healthcare is self-care, identify specific, reliable medical Internet sites both general and of the relevant specialty, and encourage your patients to use them.
- Provide for continuity of care for your patients 24 hours a day, seven days a week.
- Utilize the medical-team approach to patient care.
- Install and use a comprehensive electronic medical record system in your practice, including e-prescribing, e-mail interactions with your patients, and electronic personal health records.

Notes

1. George D. Lundberg, Chapter 11, in *Severed Trust: Why American Medicine Hasn't Been Fixed,* (New York: Basic Books, 2002).

2. Samuel Johnson. *Life of Johnson,* Vol. I. (1734; reprinted by Classic Literature Library), p. 175. Available: http://www.classic-literature.co.uk/scottish-authors/james-boswell/life-of-johnson-vol_01/ebook-page-175.asp (Accessed: April 21, 2006).

3. William M. Silberg, George D. Lundberg, and Robert A. Musacchio, "Assessing, Controlling, and Assuring the Quality of Medical Information on the Internet: Caveat Lector et Viewor—Let the Reader and the Viewer Beware," *Journal of the American Medical Association* 277 (1997): 1244–1245.

4. For example, critics of current medical publishing practices argue that the inclusion of honorary authors and ghost authors on many articles undermines the integrity of the authorship system. See A. Flanagin, L. A. Carey, P. B. Fontanarosa, S. G. Phillips, B. P. Pace, G. D. Lundberg, and D. Rennie, "Prevalence of Articles with Honorary Authors and Ghost Authors in Peer-Reviewed Medical Journals," *Journal of the American Medical Association* 280 (1998): 222–224.

5. Mohan Dutta-Bergman, "Trusted Online Sources of Health Information: Differences in Demographics, Health Beliefs, and Health-Information Orientation," *Journal of Medical Internet Research* 5 (2003): e21.

11

Trustworthy Information:
The Role of the Media

TRUDY LIEBERMAN

Can the media be trusted to provide accurate, reliable information about health and healthcare? In some cases the answer is surely yes. There are plenty of good, hardworking reporters on the healthcare beat, and there are some media outlets that print or broadcast the stories that these reporters produce. But in too many cases the answer is no. The media not only do not reinforce trust in healthcare, they actively undermine it. Media outlets fail to provide readers or viewers with the accurate information they need, and they provide too much information that is misleading, unreliable, or simply useless. This happens in identifiable ways and for understandable, if not laudable, reasons.[1]

Consider first the various pressures and influences on the media that help undermine trust. One is obviously the pressure to get the news out first, to get a scoop. Another is simply the urge to climb on the latest bandwagon. Both pressures could be seen at work a few years ago when the drug Celebrex, a COX-2 inhibitor, was released by Searle. (Searle later merged with Pharmacia; Pfizer produces the drug today.) Reporters at the press conference where the drug was introduced called in their stories on cell phones to be first with the news. Others filed their stories as quickly as they could. Few of these early stories noted any issues or concerns about the drug.[2] Almost no one, for example, mentioned a study at the University of Pennsylvania that raised questions of possible cardiac problems with all the COX-2 drugs, including Celebrex. The drug manufacturer had funded this study, but for obvious reasons, it wasn't discussed in the press release announcing Celebrex.

Driven in part by these stories, Celebrex became one of the fastest selling drugs in history. Later, of course, some patients began suffering side effects and learned that the drug may have been prescribed inappropriately. That led to questions about whether their doctors could be trusted, but it also raised concerns about whether they could trust the media coverage. As it turns out, the media did a very bad job covering the COX-2 drugs. As I documented in the July 2005

Columbia Journalism Review, the press missed many clues about the potential safety problems with Vioxx, Merck's answer to Celebrex. By the time Merck pulled the drug from the market in September 2004, as many as 140,000 Americans had suffered heart attacks due to the drug. Journalists were more interested in touting the COX-2 drugs as super aspirin than in investigating the mounting clues that the drug was unsafe. When the media hype research studies that essentially promote new drugs and gloss over or omit potential side effects or harms, the public has reason not to trust them. One reporter who works for a large metropolitan daily in the South told me that his editors always pressured him to put a positive spin on a drug at the beginning of the story. The drawbacks came much later, if at all. He added that there was pressure to get his work featured on page one, and sometimes leaving out the crucial nuances was the way to win with editors. A drug called Aricept, marketed by Pfizer, is another case in point. In the spring of 2005, the *New England Journal of Medicine* published a study about how vitamin E and the drug affected patients who had mild cognitive impairment. The study concluded that vitamin E did not forestall Alzheimer's disease, the drug did not slow progression of the disease after three years, but it did have a little bit of an effect after one year of treatment. ABC News didn't report the study results that way. Instead, both its morning and evening shows focused on the one-year effect, making it sound like a breakthrough, which it was not. The network's own journalist-doctor even recommended that people take the drug, although the *New England Journal of Medicine* study, on which the network based its segments, did not support such a clear-cut recommendation. What is the public to believe when it hears "news" like this? Such coverage, however, probably made Pfizer very happy.[3] Another pressure, less well known outside the ranks of the media, is the influence of think tanks and other ideologically driven organizations that have risen to prominence in the last 20 years. The most effective of these organizations have been on the conservative end of the political spectrum. They have had a substantial effect on how healthcare stories in the media are framed, what is reported, and what is missing from a story. [4]

An example is the selling of the Medicare budget cuts in 1997. Republicans in Congress and their allies in the think tanks wanted to change Medicare into a more privatized system, a system that more resembled the federal employees' insurance plan. They also wanted to cut the Medicare budget, which they succeeded in doing. But since Medicare is a highly popular program, they faced a problem in selling their proposals to the general public. Consequently, they attempted to disguise what was really happening. Republican operatives, notably the chairman of the Republican National Committee, Haley Barbour, met with journalists and urged them to avoid the word "cut" in their stories. Journalists tried hard to comply. If you examine the transcripts and clips of stories from that period, you see reporters stumbling over their words, trying not to say that the Republicans in Congress were cutting Medicare. A CBS reporter, for instance, was detailing the problems Medicare was facing and discussing the fact that seniors might be expected to pay more in the future. Yet she said, "It all adds up to a savings of $270 billion in the growth of Medicare spending." In fact, the $270 billion was roughly the amount that Congress had *cut* from Medicare—a cut that has since resulted in reductions in Medicare HMO drug benefits for many seniors and higher premiums. Again, readers and viewers could not rely on newspapers and television news programs to give them accurate information, so that they could voice their opinions about what was happening.

Another pressure on the news media reflects the way reporters are trained and expected to write their stories. This pressure comes from their culture, the way journalists look at things. An example is the coverage in the summer 2002 of congressional debate over adding a prescription drug benefit to Medicare. For a story published in the *Columbia Journalism Review,* I examined 127 stories from major newspapers about this debate, looking at whether the articles concentrated on the political angle—who was for it, who was against it—or on the human angle, meaning the effect of the proposed legislation on the people it was designed to benefit. The vast majority of stories concentrated on the political angle. Reporters piled quote upon quote from Democrats, Republicans, the Speaker of the House, and the leaders of the Senate and offered various prognostications about which political party would benefit more, if the drug bill were passed or if it were killed. What they did not examine was how the bill would have helped the people who needed it most.

In general, more and more media—particularly television news programs— go to great lengths to prescribe exactly what they want guests to say. A guest on the *Today* show, for example, is told what questions the hosts will ask and is given a chance to prepare her answers. But there is virtually no give and take. One foundation executive told me that she was asked to appear on the *McNeil-Lehrer News Hour* and talk about a prescription drug benefit for Medicare. The producers of the show wanted her to say that wholesale reform of Medicare was a necessary precondition for implementing a prescription drug benefit. She protested that this was not the case. Suddenly, she found herself uninvited to appear on the show.

The Vanishing Line between "Church" and "State"

Newspapers and television networks have always been commercial enterprises, and traditionally there has been a wall of sorts between the editorial side, the "church," and the publishing side, the "state." People on both sides worked hard to assure editorial independence. Granted, they didn't always succeed. I remember working as a young consumer reporter for the *Detroit Free Press* in 1968, and at first I was given a good deal of freedom to explore both the federal and the state landscape of consumer problems and legislation. At the time, incredible as it may seem, women were viewed by banks and other lenders as poor credit risks because they were likely to become pregnant and leave the workforce. Hence, they rarely were able to get credit cards in their own names. Some lobbyists and legislators in Michigan wanted to pass a law that would allow women to have their own credit. Many banks, retailers, and other industry people opposed it. I wrote an article about how certain state senators were plotting with industry interests to scuttle the idea. The article was published, but soon after I was severely chastised by the city editor, who told me that readers didn't care about what the governor or legislators were doing in Lansing, and that I should avoid writing such stories. I have often wondered how he knew that readers were not interested in this subject. My suspicion is that it had less to do with readers than with the large banks that advertised regularly in the newspaper. The city editor did not want to alienate them.

Today, unfortunately, such breaches of the "church-state" wall are no longer rare, and it is therefore much harder for readers to trust what they read in newspapers and magazines or see on television. There is a blurring between the editorial side and the business side of many, many media outlets. Not long ago, for example, a reporter from a large newspaper said to me, "You know, health is very important to us. We just had a meeting about it the other day to see how we could generate more revenue from health and medical stories." In the past, no one on the editorial side would have been concerned with generating more revenue. The two sides were more or less balanced, with the revenue needs of the newspaper matched against the public's need for reliable, unbiased information. Today the scale has been tilted, and the revenue needs of the media outweigh the information needs of the public. We have to look no further than the direct-to-consumer pharmaceutical advertising phenomenon that has emerged since the late 1990s. Media organizations benefit greatly from such advertising. In 1999, the five networks, including CNN and Fox News, received $569 million in drug company advertising revenues. By 2004, according to TNS Media Intelligence, that amount had tripled to nearly $1.5 billion.[5] Advertising revenue from drug companies to print publications is less but still significant. In 2004, drug companies spent $67 million at *Time*, $43 million at *Newsweek*, and $13 million at the *New York Times*. With so much money now at stake, how can the consumer be sure they are getting truthful and complete information? The answer is they can't.[6]

Examples of this imbalance can be found everywhere. For example, a colleague of mine who suffers from fibroid tumors was listening to radio station WCBS in New York City and was particularly interested to hear a segment about her condition. A doctor from Westchester Medical Center was discussing a treatment, and my colleague listened closely. At the end of the segment, the station aired an advertisement for the Westchester Medical Center. My colleague had no way of knowing whether what she had just heard was an independent report or a sort of infomercial and thus had no way of assessing how reliable the information was. She did not know whom she could trust.

To offer another example, I wrote an article for *Columbia Journalism Review* about NBC News.[7] NBC was one of the first media outlets to run stories about a new imaging device called the Ultrafast CT scanner, which is designed to detect calcium buildup in the coronary arteries. The stories were favorable; they focused on the great things that the new device could do, without mentioning that not all physicians shared this enthusiasm for the value of the device. In researching the article, I learned not only that NBC is owned by the same corporate parent, General Electric Co., as G.E. Medical, an $8 billion division that makes diagnostic imaging devices, but also that G.E. Medical was negotiating with Imatron, the maker of the new scanner, to market the product. (The deal was signed shortly after the broadcast.) Of course, none of this was disclosed in any of the segments. How can viewers trust NBC's information when nothing is disclosed about possible conflicts of interest? Most of the media tend to write positive articles about companies, products, and people, and in healthcare these stories typically follow a well-worn formula. Mary Smith had a problem. Dr. Jones found a solution. Readers or viewers get information about a new test, a new medicine, or whatever, but no one really knows what the evidence says about whether it is useful or not. Nor do the reporters ask fundamental questions about what problems may arise. Plenty of them wrote articles about ThinPrep, for instance, which is a new technique for testing for cervical cancer through Pap smears. But they never asked a key question, namely, What is the number of false positives generated by the new technique? Positive articles that ignore questions such as these help generate revenue for the media outlet that publishes them. The articles can be packaged as reprints and sold to the featured company. There is no additional revenue to be gleaned from negative articles. This is a message that reporters pick up on pretty quickly.

The Flood of "Expert" Advice

"Experts" seem to make an appearance in virtually every story about health-related subjects, and this journalistic device is another trust buster. Many so-called experts hardly qualify as experts; they simply may be journalists who have covered a health story or two. Many experts are invisible—they are not even identified. And some of the experts may have their own agenda. The magazine *Better Homes and Gardens,* for instance, published an article about the same Ultrafast CT. It, too, was a positive article about ultrafast scanning and how it could help prevent coronary artery disease. Among the experts quoted was an Atlanta cardiologist, who described the device as a "very promising technology" and disparaged competing diagnostic approaches such as the treadmill test. Accompanying the article was a list of 36 places around the country that offered Ultrafast CT. The Atlanta cardiologist was associated with one of them, as I later discovered, yet the article never revealed the connection. Was the expert dispassionate, or was he just trying to sell his imaging center's services?

Readers and viewers are hard put to know which experts to trust. I like to think that the magazine I work for, *Consumer Reports,* can be relied on as an expert in areas where it has conducted its usual extensive research. But should we also trust *U.S. News & World Report* for its well-known rankings of hospitals? Should we trust a regional magazine that publishes a story about the "10 best" hospitals in its area for heart by-pass surgery? Providers are disseminating their own information; so are state governments, which have weighed in with rankings based on HEDIS (Health Plan Employer Data and Information Set) scores, which measure dimensions of health quality such as whether diabetics have received eye and foot exams. The effect may be a kind of expert overload, which in the end imparts little real information. That may be beneficial: patients may eventually trust their doctor more because they trust everybody else less. But it also may lead to a kind of cognitive dissonance. If the doctor you have chosen for your heart surgery is not showing up well in the Pennsylvania Health Care Cost Containment Council's report on good cardiac doctors, what do you do? Are you really going to shop around for another cardiac specialist—especially if you need the operation right away?

Of course, journalists often assume the role of experts. A particularly insidious form of journalist-as-expert is known as "tip" journalism. It is more and more common in both newspapers and television shows: the five things you need to do to stay healthy; the three things to check before you enter a hospital; the six things to look for in a pediatrician; and so on. Tip journalism is relatively new, and I feel that journalists often rely on tips instead of doing the reporting necessary to present a well-rounded story. If a reporter can offer three tips, the editor is satisfied, the public is "informed," most advertisers are not bothered, and reporters can quickly write tips for the next story.

If you were inclined to create a taxonomy of this abhorrent species, you might classify tips into three categories. The first could be called stupid and useless. Some years back I was working on an article about nursing homes, and I visited perhaps 65 of them. Talking to a long-term-care ombudsman in a Maryland county, I was handed a pamphlet with tips on choosing a nursing home. One of the tips was, Does the patient's room enter onto a hallway? In all the nursing homes I visited, I had never seen rooms that didn't enter onto a hallway. It was like saying, Does the nursing home have a roof? If you need advice of that sort, finding a nursing home is not your biggest problem.

The second category of tips are those that pose a question to the reader or viewer without providing an answer. The fields of medicine and health seem to have many in this category. One tip that I saw, for example, urges people to find out how the doctors in their HMO are paid. I have written enough on this subject to qualify as something of an expert myself, and I have no idea how HMO doctors are paid. There are bonuses. There are withholds. Some of the compensation is based on fees for services performed, some on capitation, and so on. What is an ordinary patient to make of this? Even if your doctor can explain how he or she is paid for every service offered, which might be taxing enough, the information is not necessarily going to be helpful. Most HMO members know that plan doctors have some incentives. Whether the incentives work for patients or against them, or indeed whether they matter at all, is rarely clear. Another tip I came across urged people to search the news. Business news about your potential providers can be telling. Telling about what? Profits? Revenues? Mergers? And what are you supposed to do with the information?

And then there is the third category of tips, which boils down to do your homework and shop around. Now, there are times when that is valid advice. When an interest rate must be disclosed, for instance, it is worth knowing the difference between an auto loan at 6 percent and one at 8 percent. But in healthcare? Imagine a senior citizen attempting to shop for the Medicare HMO that has the best drug benefit. An organization in California known as the California Healthcare Foundation has teamed up with Consumers Union and has employed an actuary to find out which health plans in California have the best drug benefits. The actuary uses complex mathematical formulas and is able to produce an answer. Very few people could do this on their own. Outside of California, the information probably does not even exist. Say that one plan has a cap of $1,500 a year and doesn't cover brand-name drugs, while another has a cap of $1,300 and only covers generics, and the two have slightly different co-pays—which one is best? Shopping around isn't going to accomplish much if you can't figure out the difference between competing products.

In sum, I believe James Carey said it best. Carey, a professor at the Columbia School of Journalism, zeroed in on where the media go wrong and why they seem to undermine trust so much:

> We have a journalism that reports the continuing stream of expert opinion. But because there is no agreement among the experts, it is more like observing talk show gossip and petty manipulation than bearing witness to the truth. We have a journalism of fact without regard to understanding through which the public is immobilized and demobilized and merely ratifies judgments of the experts delivered from on high.
>
> It is a journalism that justifies itself in the public's name, but in which the public plays no role except as an audience. A receptacle to be informed by key experts and an excuse for the practice of publicity.[8]

In this environment, the question keeps circling back to whom we can trust. In healthcare, unfortunately, the public too often cannot trust the media.

Notes

1. For a discussion of the typical causes of distortions, see Jay A. Winston, "Science and the Media: The Boundaries of Truth," *Health Affairs* 4 (January 1985): 5–23, esp. 8–10.

2. Trudy Lieberman, "New Drugs: A Dose of Reality," *Columbia Journalism Review* 38 (September/October 1999): 10–11.

3. Trudy Lieberman, "Bitter Pill," *Columbia Journalism Review* 4 (July/August 2005): 45–51.

4. For a detailed discussion of the power of conservative ideologues to shape media content, see Trudy Lieberman, *Slanting the Story: The Forces that Shape the News* (New York: The New Press, 1999).

5. Lieberman, "Bitter Pill."

6. Lieberman, "Bitter Pill."

7. Trudy Lieberman, "Covering Medical Technology: The Seven Deadly Sins," *Columbia Journalism Review* 40 (September/October 2001): 24–28.

8. James Carey, "Journalists Just Leave—The Ethics of an Anomalous Profession," in *Media and Morality* , ed. Robert M. Baird, William E. Loges, and Stuart E. Rosenbaum (Amherst, N.Y.: Prometheus Books, 1999), 39–54.

12

Confusion at the Table: Can We Trust That Our Food Is Healthy?

WALTER C. WILLETT

In an industrial society, eating is necessarily an act of trust. Few of us are directly engaged in farming or food production, so we must trust that those who are will provide us with healthy foodstuffs. Then, too, most food undergoes a tremendous amount of processing, packaging, transportation, and storage before it reaches our table, and there are many things that can go wrong at each step. Yet, we cannot worry about all the dire possibilities every time we put something in our mouths. We trust that everything will be done properly and that every bite will be safe.

Sometimes, of course, this trust seems misplaced. Newspapers and television news shows periodically report on microbial contamination of food, such as outbreaks of *E. coli* infection and other sorts of food poisoning. The Centers for Disease Control (CDC) report that somewhere between 5,000 and 10,000 deaths occur each year because of food poisoning. But the trust problems go even deeper than this. In all likelihood, hundreds of thousands of additional deaths occur each year because people are eating food that is not optimally healthy for them. Worse, many of these people are following the dietary advice of their physicians, the government, or some other authority. Think of all the people in the past couple of decades who were advised to switch from butter to margarine, for example. As it turns out, that was probably not very good advice.

This chapter focuses on a question that is central to the maintenance of trust: To what extent can we or should we trust the recommendations about food that are periodically handed down by the government and other organizations? We look at the issue of *trans*-fatty acids, which provides an excellent example of the complexities involved in this area and of the dangers of making strong statements without strong scientific evidence.

The Food Pyramid and Trans Fats

The U.S. Department of Agriculture's (USDA) food pyramid may be the most recognized icon of nutritional advice anywhere. It appears on the back of breakfast cereal boxes. It is used in schools to teach children healthy nutrition. Surveys indicate that the vast majority of Americans recognize it. At the bottom of the original pyramid used from 1992 to 2005 was the category "Bread, Cereal, Rice, and Pasta Groups," with a daily recommendation of six to 11 servings. One rung up was the vegetable group (three to five servings) and fruit group (two to four servings), and above them were Milk, Yogurt, and Cheese, and Meat, Poultry, Fish, Dry Beans, Eggs, and Nuts (two to three servings each). At the very top were Fats, Oils, and Sweets, with the sole recommendation to use sparingly.

The main message of the original food pyramid, in short, was that all fats are bad. Carbohydrates, by contrast, are good. They were the foundation of the food pyramid, and we were told that we could eat up to 11 servings a day (plus potatoes,

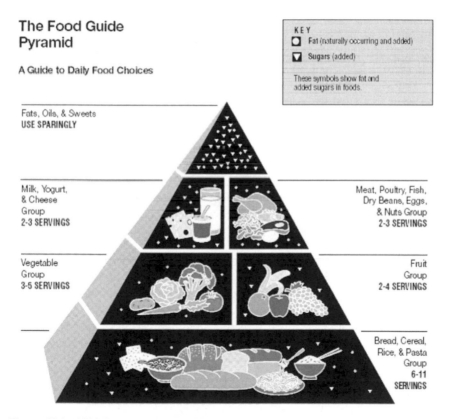

Figure 12.1. 1992 Food Guide Pyramid

Source: U.S. Department of Agriculture, *The Food Guide Pyramid,* Home and Garden Bulletin No. 252 (Washington, D.C.: U.S. Government Printing Office, 1992).

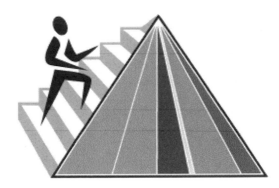

Figure 12.2. 2005 Food Guide Pyramid

Source: U.S. Department of Agriculture, Center for Nutrition Policy and Promotion, April 2005. Available: http://www.mypyramid.gov/ (accessed April 19, 2006).

which are included in the vegetable group).[1] In 2005, the USDA issued a new pyramid of colored stripes that failed to convey any information about foods to be emphasized or eaten sparingly. Persons with sufficient motivation and resources could find detailed and complex information on the USDA MyPyramid website (http://www.mypyramid.gov).

The original USDA food pyramid admonition to avoid fat and emphasize carbohydrates reflected the general views of the nutrition community from the late 1980s until very recently. For example, the American Heart Association offered advice about how to substitute low-fat or nonfat products for high-fat ones (e.g., nonfat solid dressings, fat-free cookies and crackers). But is it really good to eat very little fat and lots of carbohydrates? Articles in the popular press periodically raise this question and often suggest that diets such as the Atkins diet—high in protein and fat, low in carbohydrates—might be better after all. Because the scientific community seems to be flip-flopping, the public scarcely knows what to believe. Indeed, surveys reveal a great deal of confusion about nutrition, including the belief that perhaps what you eat really does not matter at all for your health.

This is a shame, because in fact the scientific community for some years now has been coming up with results supporting some very clear recommendations. In 1987, my colleagues Ronald Mensink and Martijn Katan studied a group of people who had been eating a traditional Western diet, in which 40 percent of the calories are supplied by fat.[2] They divided these people into two groups. One group replaced 10 percent of its saturated fat calories with complex carbohydrates, which was consistent with the American Heart Association's recommendations at the time. The other group replaced 10 percent of its saturated fat calories with olive oil, which is mainly monounsaturated fat. What they found was that total cholesterol declined about equally on these two diets. However, levels of HDL cholesterol (high-density lipoproteins, the "good" cholesterol) stayed about the same for people on the olive-oil diet and declined significantly for people on the complex-carbohydrate diet. Meanwhile, triglycerides rose on the complex-carbohydrate diet and declined slightly on the olive-oil diet. Based on these results, a person would be better off on a higher fat diet, as long as it was primarily monounsaturated fat, than on a complex-carbohydrate diet.

In the early 1990s, nutritional studies began to suggest that *trans*-fatty acids, or trans fats, had a significant influence on blood lipids such as cholesterol and triglycerides. Sometime around 1900, the food industry developed a process called partial hydrogenation, which converts liquid vegetable oils to solid fat by creating trans fat from unsaturated fats. That is how liquid corn oil is turned into products such as Crisco and margarine. Today, trans fat occurs in many manufactured food products, including virtually all commercial baked goods. Because the process destroys the essential omega-3 fatty acids that occur naturally in soybean and other plant oils, it allows for a much longer shelf life. Thanks to partial hydrogenation, baked goods can sit on a store shelf for many months.

In 1990, Drs. Mensink and Katan published a seminal paper in the *New England Journal of Medicine* examining what trans fats do to blood lipids.[3] They compared the effects of replacing unsaturated fats with either trans fats or saturated fats. The trans fat diet raised total cholesterol about half as much as the saturated fat diet, and the food industry promptly used this result to claim that trans fats were good because they led to less elevated serum cholesterol levels. The trouble was, however, that total serum cholesterol levels were not the most important figures to analyze. Trans fats depress HDL cholesterol significantly, and thereby raise the ratio of LDL (low-density lipoproteins, the "bad" cholesterol) to HDL substantially more than saturated fat does. The result is a substantially worse lipid profile. This finding has been confirmed in many studies, which have also confirmed that trans fats have many other deleterious effects, such as increasing blood triglycerides and lipoprotein (a) levels, adversely affecting endothelial function and probably increasing insulin resistance as well.

An Empirical Basis for Dietary Guidance

Lipid levels are important in overall health, but there are many other pathways by which dietary changes could influence the risk for cardiovascular disease. To evaluate the effects of other changes, our group has set up long-term studies of very large populations. The intent is to assess the clinical endpoint, not simply one or another intermediate biochemical variable. The Nurses Health Study, for example, has followed 121,700 female nurses over a period of more than 25 years, beginning in 1976. The Health Professionals Follow-Up Study, begun in 1986, focuses on 52,000 male health professionals. The Nurses Health Study II began in 1989 and has followed 116,000 nurses. The rationale of these large studies was to create an empirical basis for dietary advice and decision making. We found in the late 1970s that people were being given a lot of advice without much data to support it. They were told to avoid eggs, for instance, yet there never has been a study showing that people who ate more eggs had more heart attacks. The large studies also provide repeated measurements over a long period of time. This is important, because both the food supply and individual eating patterns change over time.

At any rate, the studies have provided some strong evidence about the relationship between dietary patterns and health. For example, we have examined the connection between dietary fats and heart disease and found that there was no relation between total fat and heart disease. That is because some types of fat are harmful and some types are helpful, as one would guess from their effects on blood lipids. Trans fats have proved to be the worst type of fat with regard to the risk for heart disease, but polyunsaturated fat is strongly beneficial. People who consumed large amounts of trans fat and low amounts of polyunsaturated fat had almost three times as great a risk for heart disease than those who did the opposite.[4] This is a large difference in risk.

The sad fact, moreover, is that people became high-risk candidates by following seemingly reputable dietary advice. They switched from butter to margarine, and although there are trans fat–free margarines on the market now, most margarines in the time period studied were high in trans fats. They also ate food made with vegetable fat such as Crisco, because they had learned that vegetable fats were better than animal fats. Unfortunately, Crisco is also loaded with trans fats.[5] Ironically, lard might have been a better choice—although the best choice is natural unsaturated fats. Perhaps they were also following the American Heart Association's guidelines and eating fat-free salad dressing. Unfortunately, a major source of omega-3 fatty acids in the food supply was full-fat salad dressing, because it is typically made from soybean oil, which is naturally high in omega-3 fatty acids. There is now strong evidence that omega-3 fatty acids reduce the likelihood of ventricular fibrillation and sudden death. So, women using full-fat salad dressing had about half the risk for dying from heart disease as women who rarely used it.[6]

Another sad dietary story is that people were advised to give up nuts because they are high in fat. Indeed, about 80 percent of the nutritional content in nuts is fat, but it is almost all unsaturated fat, which is beneficial. Nut consumption in the Nurses Health Study has declined by about 50 percent since the 1980s. But women who consume nuts on most days had about a 30 percent lower risk of heart attack, which is consistent with the effect of unsaturated fat on blood lipids.[7] Some people who gave up nuts thereby put themselves at higher risk, and some undoubtedly died because of it. Similarly, recent research examined nuts and the risk for type II diabetes. There, too, is about a 30 percent reduction in type II diabetes risk in people with higher consumption of nuts.

Though some of these conclusions may sound radical, they are not. A National Academy of Sciences report published in 1989 concluded that intake of total fat per se, independent of the relative content of different types of fatty acids, was not associated with high blood cholesterol and coronary heart disease.[8] And evidence has since mounted that the type of fat is very important. But even now, the food pyramid and much other dietary advice remain unchanged. People are told that they should eliminate fat entirely.

Of course, if total fat were related to other important conditions, such as a lower risk for some kind of cancer, it might still make sense to reduce one's fat intake. In fact, some researchers hypothesized that fat was strongly related to breast, colon, and prostate cancer. No data has been found in the Nurses Health Study, however, to support this hypothesis for breast or colon cancer. The association is actually weakly but significantly *inverse;* the highest risks are actually among women with the lowest fat intake.[9] The general lack of association has been confirmed by several other large studies as well.

The Truth about Carbohydrates

Most of the attention on diet in the popular media has been focused on fat. Reducing fat seems to be the main point of the government's food pyramid and of other advice, such as that from the American Heart Association. But just in the last few years, both reputable and not-so-reputable purveyors of nutritional advice have begun to focus on the adverse effect of high levels of carbohydrates in a diet. Interestingly, this is an area that has been largely neglected by nutritional science, despite the fact that carbohydrates are the major sources of calories in almost all diets.

What we do know, however, is that there are important differences among carbohydrates that have not been widely acknowledged or appreciated. One category of carbohydrate is known as high glycemic or easily digested carbohydrate. A bagel is a perfect example. People have been told that a bagel is a healthy choice because it is fat free. But when you eat a bagel, your body rapidly breaks down the starch, converts it to blood glucose, and your blood glucose rises sharply. Since the body does not want high levels of blood glucose, the pancreas puts out a blast of insulin. The glucose declines sharply, and three or four hours later, many people are hypoglycemic.

This rapid rise and decline in blood sugar can have serious adverse effects. The rapid decline usually makes people hungry. So they tend to snack and take in extra calories. These large increases in blood glucose are related to the elevation of triglycerides and reduction in HDL cholesterol, which could add to the risk for heart disease. Finally, it is possible that repeated demand for high insulin output over the years can lead to what is now recognized as pancreatic exhaustion. That is the point at which an individual develops type II diabetes.

A second category of carbohydrates, in contrast, is called low-glycemic carbohydrate. It is characterized by slower digestion, slower absorption, and less increase in blood glucose. These carbohydrates include whole grains, such as whole-wheat pasta and brown rice. Because they take longer to digest, they are unlikely to lead to hunger and snacking between meals. Whole-grain, high-fiber carbohydrates can have a positive effect on health outcomes when consumed in moderation. In the Nurses Health Study, for example, we found that women who ate the lowest amounts of low-glycemic, high-fiber cereal grains had a risk for type II diabetes about two-and-a-half times that of women who ate the most.[10] Here again, the women in the high-risk category had followed the recommendations in the USDA pyramid. They were told, in effect, to eat bagels, bread, and pasta, maybe with a fat-free sauce. They were told to eat fat-free yogurt for dessert or perhaps some fat-free cookies or cakes. Unfortunately, that kind of diet helped land them in the high-risk category.

Weight itself, of course, is a very important predictor of health outcomes. The problems associated with obesity—a body mass index (BMI) of over 30— are well known. But even with BMIs in the 20-to-30 range, the data show a strong gradient associating weight with adverse outcomes. For example, between 18.5 and 25 BMI, there is more than a fivefold gradient of increasing risk for type II diabetes.[11] The standard advice to people who are obese or overweight has been to get the fat out of their diet. Unfortunately, the few studies that have examined this recommendation do not support it. To be sure, most studies show short-term weight reductions in people who are put on a low-fat diet. But when these people return for follow-up a year or more later, the weight has almost always returned. In well-designed randomized trials that have continued for a year or more, not one has shown a reduction in weight due to a low-fat diet. The recommendation to eliminate fat is simply not effective for long-term weight control. It is another example of "scientific" advice that is not supported by good science.

We have seen the many potential problems with the advice conveyed by the USDA food pyramid in its original form. Still, no one until recently had studied whether people who follow that pyramid over the long run did better or worse in terms of overall health. Marjorie McCullough, while a doctoral student in our nutritional epidemiology program, did just this. She utilized what is known as the Healthy Eating Index (HEI), which the Department of Agriculture used as a way to score diets according to their adherence to the dietary pyramid and U.S. dietary guidelines. (Essentially, an individual receives points for eating or avoiding items on the pyramid in the prescribed proportions.) The long-term studies provided massive amounts of dietary data, and we were able to calculate HEI figures for more than 100,000 men and women. Then we looked at major chronic diseases as the outcome: any cancer, any heart attack, any stroke, and other nontraumatic cause of death.

When the data were adjusted only for age, there was a significant relationship; that is, the higher an individual scored on the HEI, the lower was the risk for major chronic disease. But since people who do what they are told about diet also tend to have good lifestyle habits (e.g., not smoking, exercising, etc.), it was also important to control for these variables. When we did so, we found that there was essentially no relationship between HEI scores and major chronic disease. This conclusion held up for both sexes.[12]

When we published this study, some people concluded that diet did not really matter for health at all. We did not believe that was an appropriate conclusion, so we created an alternative healthy eating index that took into account types of fat, types of carbohydrates, and sources of protein. For example, there is much evidence that fish, chicken, and nuts are healthier sources of protein than large amounts of red meat. The alternative healthy eating index did show a major benefit in reducing the risk for cardiovascular disease, but not much of a benefit in reducing cancer risk. Staying lean and being physically active are both important in terms of reducing cancer incidence, and there are individual relationships between certain types of cancers and certain foods. But overall in this study, the impact of diet on cancer risk was not substantial.[13]

Of course, we do not now know all the truth about the relationship between diet and health. Research will continue, and scientists will produce more refined findings. The point is that in the past, scientists and nutritionists have given strong advice that was not well supported by evidence. Positions often changed radically, seemingly capriciously, and the public felt betrayed. Our ability to provide guidance is certainly much better now than it was 20 years ago. Unfortunately, there is a legacy of mistrust from the past 20 years that we will have to overcome.

Notes

1. U.S. Department of Agriculture, *The Food Guide Pyramid,* Home and Garden Bulletin No. 252 (Washington, D.C.: U.S. Government Printing Office, 1992).

2. R. P. Mensink and M. B. Katan, "Effect of Monounsaturated Fatty Acids versus Complex Carbohydrates on High-Density Lipoprotein in Healthy Men and Women," *Lancet* 1 (1987): 122–125.

3. R. P. Mensink and M. B. Katan, "Effect of Dietary *Trans*-Fatty Acids on High-Density and Low-Density Lipoprotein Cholesterol Levels in Healthy Subjects," *New England Journal of Medicine* 323 (1990): 439–445.

4. F. B. Hu, M. J. Stampfer, J. E. Manson et al., "Dietary Fat Intake and the Risk of Coronary Heart Disease in Women," *New England Journal of Medicine* 337 (1997): 1491–1499.

5. Crisco was only very recently introduced to the market in a in a trans fat–free version.

6. F. B. Hu, M. J. Stampfer, J. E. Manson et al., "Dietary Intake of α-Linolenic Acid and Risk of Fatal Ischemic Heart Disease among Women," *American Journal of Clinical Nutrition* 69 (1999): 890–897.

7. F. B. Hu, M. J. Stampfer, J. E. Manson et al., "Frequent Nut Consumption and Risk of Coronary Heart Disease in Women: Prospective Cohort Study," *British Medical Journal* 317 (1998): 1341–1345.

8. National Research Council (U.S.), Committee on Diet and Health, *Diet and Health: Implications for Reducing Chronic Disease Risk* (Washington, D.C.: National Academy Press, 1989).

9. M. D. Holmes, D. J. Hunter, G. A. Colditz et al., "Association of Dietary Intake of Fat and Fatty Acids with Risk of Breast Cancer," *Journal of the American Medical Association* 281 (1999): 914–920.

10. J. Salmeron, J. E. Manson, M. J. Stampfer, G. A. Colditz, A.L. Wing, and W. C. Willett, "Dietary Fiber, Glycemic Load, and Risk of Non–Insulin-Dependent Diabetes Mellitus in Women," *Journal of the American Medical Association* 277 (1997): 472–477.

11. W. C. Willett, W. H. Dietz, and G. A. Colditz, "Guidelines for Healthy Weight," *New England Journal of Medicine* 341 (1999): 427–434.

12. M. L. McCullough, D. Feskanich, E. B. Rimm et al., "Adherence to the *Dietary Guidelines for Americans* and Risk of Major Chronic Disease in Men," *American Journal of Clinical Nutrtition* 72 (2000): 1223–1231.

13. M. L. McCullough, D. Feskanich, M. J. Stampfer et al., "Diet Quality and Major Chronic Disease Risk in Men and Women: Moving toward Improved Dietary Guidance," *American Journal of Clinical Nutrition* 76 (2002): 1261–1271.

13

Trust in Vaccines

MARIE C. McCORMICK

Ever since Dr. Edward Jenner developed his vaccine against smallpox, immunization has been perceived as one of the great triumphs of medical science over infectious disease. To be sure, not everyone accepted this triumph; small minorities of the population in the United States and many other countries have always mistrusted vaccines, just as they have always mistrusted science. But until quite recently, it seemed that mistrust of immunization was a sort of cultural lag, an old-fashioned and uninformed belief that would die out as people saw that immunizations were effective in preventing disease.

In the last decade or so, however, mistrust of immunizations has increased, particularly with regard to the childhood immunization schedule. Growing numbers of parents express concern about the safety and effectiveness of vaccines for their children. As the vaccination goals for children under five for the Healthy People 2010 project were exceeded sooner than expected, in 2005, apparently this concern has not resulted in a lower vaccination rate.[1] However, parents seem to have more questions and require more persuasion to vaccinate their children. Web sites and books trumpet the alleged (and sometimes real) failings and abuses of vaccines and the immunization process, to the point where even people who believe in medical science may feel confused. This chapter traces this decline of trust by describing and analyzing a handful of trust busters—developments that have sown confusion and doubt in the minds of many. It also examines several ways by which the medical and professional communities can enhance trust in vaccines and immunization.

Trust Busters

Where vaccines are concerned, the decline in trust can be traced to changes of policy, to adverse events, to myths, to the spread of misinformation, and to poorly designed or incomplete scientific research. Each of these trust busters alone might provoke a few nagging doubts even in otherwise well-informed people. As a group, however, they have created a climate of mistrust that seems to permeate much public debate on the subject.

Changes in Policy

Vaccine policy regarding which vaccines should be administered to whom and under what conditions changes over time. But change is always threatening, even more so when it is poorly managed. Not long ago, the childhood immunization schedule consisted of only a few vaccines, such as DPT (diphtheria-pertussis-tetanus) and polio. Today, it typically includes vaccines against 11 infectious agents. This expansion of the schedule may not be well received by parents; indeed, some 25 percent of parents in a recent survey responded that "too many" immunizations are being given to their children and that these vaccines might actually weaken the child's immune system.[2]

In recent years, some rather abrupt changes have been made in vaccine policy for safety reasons. Rotavirus vaccine was introduced, but it was quickly discontinued when it was associated with intussusception.[3] Thimerosal, the mercury-based preservative used in vaccines until a few years ago, was removed as a precaution to reduce exposure to all types of mercury.[4] These changes left people saying to their physicians and public health officials, in effect, You told me last year that these vaccines were safe, and today you're taking them off the market—when am I going to believe you? It doesn't help matters that some observers think that members of the official panels making recommendations about the vaccine schedule may not be completely disinterested in the decisions. The panels include people who develop the vaccines and therefore may have some interest in seeing them used. They also include people from the large pharmaceutical manufacturers. While, clearly, such individuals have significant expertise of the sort needed to make recommendations, it is not clear to the public that these panels are without conflicts of interest.

Adverse Events

Adverse vaccine events are situations in which an individual is injured or dies as a result of immunization. These trust busters may be an inescapable part of any large-scale immunization program; no vaccine is 100 percent safe, and in a large population even a tiny percentage of adverse events adds up to a significant number. When the government requires a vaccine for children, it also exposes them to the risk for an adverse event. This naturally sits poorly with many parents. Then, too, vaccine manufacturers are exempted from legal risk. If a child experiences a recognized adverse event, the family may receive compensation from the Justice Department, but they may not sue the vaccine's manufacturer. In that event, people often feel that they are deprived of their legal rights.

The Centers for Disease Control and Prevention (CDC), of course, maintain an adverse-event reporting program, known as VAERS (Vaccine Adverse Event Reporting System), which is accessible to everyone. The pharmaceutical companies maintain a postmarketing surveillance system. Neither of these safeguards is seen as entirely satisfactory. People who notify authorities of an adverse event often feel that they receive little response, in part because of the necessary triaging of reports to focus on the more serious ones. They notice that the same agency, the CDC, is responsible both for setting policy and for examining adverse events. (These are the responsibilities of two separate groups within the CDC, but lay people do not know about or may not trust that the groups act independently.) Moreover, adverse events occur in the context of a lack of experience with the wild-type disease. Many parents and doctors, even some grandparents, have never seen a case of measles or other vaccine-preventable diseases. As a result, they do not understand the nature of the adverse events that are associated with the disease.

Myths about Vaccines

The CDC has identified several widespread myths about vaccines. One is that preventable diseases were already on the decline before the advent of large-scale immunization programs. For a few diseases, such as diphtheria, this is indeed the case. For many others, such as hemophilus or polio, it is far from the case. A second myth is that most people who now contract a disease have already been immunized. Again, there is some truth to this: if a vaccine is only 90 percent effective, for example, 10 percent of those who are immunized will be susceptible to the disease.

A third myth is that preventable diseases have been eradicated in the United States.[5] Again, this is true in isolated instances, such as measles. To paraphrase Mexican public health expert Dr. Julio Frenk, the longest plane ride is shorter than the incubation period of any infectious disease. While a disease may not occur naturally in the United States, it can certainly be imported. And a fourth myth is that there are so-called hot lots of vaccine. This myth is derived from the fact that the adverse-event reporting system shows that some vaccine lots lead to more adverse events than others do. Because it is considered proprietary information, manufacturers are not required to report the number of a hot lot actually in the field. So we do not know the ratio of adverse events to inoculations from any given lot. Finally, a fifth myth is that multiple immunizations cause immune dysfunction. This claim has been well studied, and it is not true.[6]

Misinformation

Thanks to the Internet, information is widely available, easily disseminated, and cheap. So is misinformation, and in the world of vaccines misinformation is rife. One site on the World Wide Web, for example, announces that immunizations may lead to a 400-fold increase in morbidity, prevent only a few cases of polio and deaths from pertussis a year, while causing thousands of cases of type 1 diabetes. The site, Vaccine Safety Website, is the work of one individual and is based on his study, which looked at the rise in diabetes cases in the United States compared to the rise in immunizations and concluded that the immunizations caused the diabetes. Nor is the site unusual in its ill-informed concerns. Other such Web sites include "Death: Vaccines; Vaccines Cause Brain Disorders in Children"; "Vaccines and Sudden Infant Death Syndrome (SIDS): A Link?"; and "Vaccines Prevent Health." The National Vaccine Information Center Website includes pathetic images of children allegedly injured by vaccines.

The Web is also a marketing medium for other forms of publication, such as books. One book, *Vaccines: A Second Opinion,* has a partial table of contents posted on the Web, which includes these chapter titles: "Vaccines Are Based on Unsound Principles," "Questionable Science," "Vaccine Propaganda," "Toxic Vaccine Ingredients," and "Vaccine Failures." Consumers Union has reviewed Web sites related to vaccines and immunization information. The organization recommends going to reliable sites like the CDC or the National Network for Immunization Information and warns that many sites are really antivaccine.[7]

Incomplete Science

I do not wish to paint a picture only of valiant but beleaguered professionals under attack by the poorly informed. Scientists and medical researchers have earned their share of the blame as well. Some studies are simply poorly designed, such as those that postulate a connection between variables that may or may not be related (e.g., immunizations and diabetes). Others jump to premature conclusions. Dr. Andrew Wakefield, a British physician, appeared on the television program *60 Minutes* to propound a theory relating autism to the measles-mumps-rubella (MMR) vaccine.[8] It was based on little more than Wakefield's having seen measles virus particles in the gastrointestinal tracts of some individuals with autism who also had gastrointestinal problems. His study describing this link, published in *Lancet,* never proved that the vaccine caused autism. Within five years, this study and Wakefield's public reservations about the vaccines resulted in vaccination rates in Great Britain falling to only 80 percent. In the United States, his study has been used to support antivaccination advocacy efforts, but vaccination rates in the United States have not fallen similarly.[9] Even though it is inconclusive, his study has had a significant impact on the debate.

Another scientific failing is lack of study. At this writing, for instance, there is very little data available on the toxicology of thimerosal. That has not stopped writers in the popular press from positing a connection between vaccines containing thimerosal and autism. Even the *New York Times* publishes this kind of shallow reporting, and it is because so little solid information was available.[10] The lack of information contributes to reasoning by analogy, which is the stock-in-trade of some groups who are suspicious of vaccines. One published paper lists the symptoms of mercury toxicity and the symptoms of autism side by side; it argues, in effect, that the symptoms are similar, ergo autism must be caused by mercury. The paper evinces no understanding of the mechanisms by which these symptoms occur, which are quite different in the two cases.[11] Since then, these and other arguments linking autism and thimerosal have been thoroughly reviewed with the conclusion that the linkage is unproven.[12]

Enhancing Trust

The medical and scientific communities obviously face a big challenge where vaccines are concerned, namely enhancing the trust with which the general public regards the entire endeavor. I believe that there are a series of steps that can help move us in that direction.

One is to enlist respected, neutral agencies to act as a kind of arbiter. After several years of controversy, in 2000 the CDC and the National Institutes of Health asked the Institute of Medicine (IOM) to establish the Institute of Medicine Immunization Safety Review Committee to examine immunization safety issues. The IOM is the medical branch of the National Academy of Sciences, a neutral, nonprofit institution created in 1863 to provide scientific advice to the government. The IOM, founded in 1970, has been involved in vaccine reporting and safety issues for a decade. So it is a perfect example of the kind of agency that is needed to undertake unbiased research and evaluation.

To enhance trust still further, the IOM established a rigorous selection process for membership on this committee. Prospective members could have no financial ties to vaccine manufacturers or their parent companies. They were allowed no past or present service on vaccine advisory committees. They were disqualified for having given expert testimony, for authoring publications on issues of vaccine safety, and for receiving current or recent funding from the CDC. The restrictions were so severe that they provoked the cynical remark that the IOM now had a whole panel of people who knew nothing about vaccines. But it was also a panel with a consistent membership committed to public health and without possible conflicts of interest. The stringent rules were considered necessary to assure the public that the reports would be neutral and untainted. I had the privilege of chairing this committee for three years. I do believe that our reports have been reassuring, at least within the professional community.

A second approach to enhancing trust entails a more proactive approach to adverse events. The current system includes three sets of clinical trials to assess safety, immunogenicity, and effectiveness before the vaccines are licensed. Once an immunization program begins, the companies conduct postmarketing surveillance, and the CDC maintains its reporting program, VAERS. But recently the CDC has begun to experiment with more proactive steps. In 2002, it set up examination centers where people who feel they have had an adverse vaccine event can receive a standardized physical examination. The CDC has entered into an agreement, called the Vaccine Safety Data Link project, with several large HMOs to use their databases to examine associations between vaccines and other health events.

A third approach is to improve access to accurate information, that is, to make it as easy for the public to find good information as it now is for them to find bad.

The Web sites of both the CDC and the FDA, for instance, have been cumbersome and difficult to use. It would help, too, if the professional community paid more attention to early identification of emerging concerns. Only recently has anyone surveyed parents to find out their current thinking regarding vaccines and how many are concerned about the vaccine schedule. No one knows precisely how large the various advocacy groups are and how representative they are of parents.

All of this, of course, is work in progress and no doubt will be for some time. Certainly, there are many issues that need further attention. We need better communication about the introduction of new vaccines and about changes to the vaccine schedule. Many professionals were roundly taken aback by the change to thimerosal-free vaccines because they did not see it coming. The composition and rationale of policymaking committees also needs to be examined, and the policy framework must be broadened to include epidemiological, ethical, and economic issues. Perhaps the very basis of vaccine policy—everybody gets everything—should be reexamined, so that people instead receive combinations of vaccines tailored to their risk factors. The public must be involved in these discussions so that all points of view are represented.[13]

Finally, the entire immunization program needs to be better understood as a case study of government-mandated risk exposure. What has happened in vaccines is similar to what happened with other exposures, such as the reactions to Agent Orange and the possible reactions to toxin exposure that may cause Gulf War syndrome. We need to know the natural history of the response to such exposures. What are the sources of discontent? Are there early-intervention points where negative responses can be met and defused to prevent escalation into confrontational tactics? What is the role of communication of risk in these settings—how do people understand it, and how do those responsible for the program get their message across? These are the sorts of questions raised in the current climate of mistrust regarding vaccines.[14] They are the questions that, in the future, require good answers.

Implications for Busy Clinicians

Those on the front line of primary care know only too well that the concern about vaccines affects their practice. Patients come in with more questions and greater reluctance to accept unquestioningly recommendations regarding immunizations. The former committee members who are also primary care providers have some advice for providers.

Provide Accurate and Reliable Information

While most parents and patients may be satisfied with relatively brief handouts, many are now searching the Web and finding far more detailed and serious concerns. Providers must be prepared to listen to these concerns and address them.

Professional societies and the CDC attempt to keep up with the emerging concerns and provide responses. The clinicians who were on our committee, however, say that our reports are invaluable, concise summaries of the scientific literature (to access the activities of the committee from 2001–2004, including the reports, see http://www.iom.edu/?ID=4705).

Be Flexible

The various vaccine advisory boards have a recommended schedule for administering vaccines, but these schedules allow some latitude to deal with clinical situations. Familiarity with the permissible variations consistent with achieving a suitable immune response may provide an opportunity for parents to accept many vaccines, while working through their concerns about one or two.

Be Patient

Over and over, parents who believe that their children were injured by vaccines—and those with ongoing concerns—tell us that they are angry about not being listened to or having their concerns addressed.[15] Willingness to address parental or patient concerns with solid information and flexibility in scheduling vaccines may help to restore trust in professionals and in the vaccine program.

Acknowledgment

This chapter represents the author's personal views and should not be construed as representing the views or recommendations of the Institute of Medicine Immunization Safety Review Committee.

Notes

1. Healthy People 2010 is a U.S. federal government–coordinated set of health objectives for the nation. The project is described and provides publications at http://www.healthypeople.gov (accessed August 8, 2005). The project's vaccine targets are available at http://www.healthypeople.gov/document/html/volume1/14Immunization.htm#_Toc4945 10242 (accessed August 8, 2005).

2. B. G. Gellin, E. W. Maibach, and E. K. Marcuse, "Do Parents Understand Immunizations? A National Telephone Survey," *Pediatrics* 106 (2000): 1097–1102.

3. M. Rennels, "The Rotavirus Vaccine Story: A Clinical Investigator's View," *Pediatrics* 106 (2000): 123–125.

4. Leslie K. Ball et al., "An Assessment of Thimerosal Use in Childhood Vaccine," *Pediatrics* 107 (May 2001): 1147–1154.

5. S. K. Obaro and A. Palmer, "Vaccines for Children: Policies, Politics, and Poverty," *Vaccine* 21 (2003): 1423–1431.

6. K. Stratton, C. B. Wilson, M. C. McCormick, eds., *Immunization Safety Review, Multiple Immunizations and Immune Dysfunction* (Washington, D.C.: National Academies Press, 2002).

7. "Vaccines: An Issue of Trust," *Consumer Reports* 66 (August 2001): 17–21.

8. *60 Minutes*, November 12, 2000.

9. J. Colgrove and R. Bayer, "Could It Happen Here? Vaccine Risk Controversies and the Specter of Derailment: A Successful Immunization System Depends Mostly on People's Willingness to Have Themselves and Their Children Vaccinated," *Health Affairs* (May-June 2005). Wakefield's 1998 study was disavowed by *The Lancet* in 2004, due to ethics and disclosure violations. See R. Horton, "A Statement by the Editors of *The Lancet,*" *The Lancet,* 363 (2004): 820–821.

10. A. Allen, "The Not-So-Crackpot Autism Theory," *New York Times Sunday Magazine,* November 10, 2002.

11. S. Bernard, A. Enayati, L. Redwood, H. Roger, and T. Binstock, "Autism: A Novel Form of Mercury Poisoning," *Medical Hypothesis* 56 (2001): 462–471.

12. Immunization Safety Review, *Vaccines and Autism* (Washington, D.C.: The National Academies Press, 2004).

13. C. Feudtner and E. K. Marcuse, "Ethics and Immunization Policy: Promoting Dialogue to Sustain Consensus," *Pediatrics* 107 (2001): 1158–1164.

14. Ayala Maayan-Metzger, Peri Kedem-Friedrich, and Jacob Kuint, "To Vaccinate or Not to Vaccinate—That Is the Question: Why Are Some Mothers Opposed to Giving Their Infants Hepatitis B. Vaccine?" *Vaccine* 23 (2005): 1941–1948.

15. For social and psychological factors and recommendations for communications improvement, see Nick Raithatha, Richard Holland, Simon Gerrard, and Ian Harvey, "A Qualitative Investigation of Vaccine Risk Perception amongst Parents Who Immunize Their Children: A Matter of Public Health Concern," *Journal of Public Health Medicine* 25 (2003): 161–164; and Leslie K. Ball, Geoffrey Evans, and Anne Bostrom, "Risky Business: Challenges in Vaccine Risk Communication," *Pediatrics* 101 (1998): 453–458.

14

Trust in the Trenches: Developing the Patient-Physician Dyad in Medical Genetics

SUSAN P. PAUKER

In the post–Human Genome Project era, delicate clinical genetic issues abound in all fields of medical practice. Medical genetics is a crucible of trust. The knowledge it provides forces patients to confront sudden, often painfully difficult decisions. The following scenarios describe the types of challenges medical genetics presents to physicians and their patients.

- Imagine that you are 43 and your second wife is 47. She is pregnant with twins. Ultrasound examination suggests that there is a one-in-ten risk for Down syndrome in one of the twins. The other twin is probably unaffected. As a couple, you have waited to start a family, and you are excited about the pregnancy—but now you find out that things are not going as planned. What do you do?
- You notice that your father has been stumbling a lot. You also notice that he is forgetful, but so are you, so you don't pay much attention to that. Then he begins to flail randomly as he walks, and you take him to the doctor. He is diagnosed with Huntington disease. You learn about this just as you are switching jobs and health insurance carriers. You also learn that you have a fifty-fifty risk of having inherited the gene that causes the disorder. If you have, you will experience the neurological degeneration that is plaguing your father. You plan to have a family. Do you want to be tested for this genetic mutation?
- You are a physician caring for an infant, and everything is going well. However, the newborn screening is positive that the baby is a carrier for cystic fibrosis (CF). The parents ask to be tested out of concern for their other children and for future pregnancies. The test results show that neither parent is a carrier for CF. You saw the infant come out of the mother. How do you raise the question of paternity?
- Your mother, her mother, and her sister all developed breast cancer prior to menopause. You have an identical twin, who wants to be tested for the breast cancer gene (BRCA) mutation. If she tests positive, you test positive as well, because you have identical genes. You will learn, with or without your consent, if you have inherited the breast cancer gene. What are your choices?

When patients learn something that may turn their life plans and expectations upside down, they rely on medical genetics clinicians to provide them with life-critical information, risk assessment, and decision support. Genetic clinicians include physician geneticists, who typically pursue a postresidency fellowship in medical genetics; Ph.D.s; nurses with advanced training in genetics; and counselors with master's degrees in human genetics. Patients must trust that those professionals will act with their best interests at heart. This chapter explores that crucible of trust. It uses the medical genetics specialty to demonstrate how practitioners can build trust into the physician-patient dyad under some of the most trying circumstances.

Understanding Medical Genetics

The field of medical genetics is growing rapidly, as knowledge of people's genetic makeup is exploding. The Human Genome Project, for instance, provides a detailed map of human DNA. The field of proteinomics studies what the gene sequencing codes determine and attempts to discover how that process works and what happens when it fails. Medical geneticists in clinical practice perform molecular, chromosomal, and metabolic tests, and of course take family histories to determine patterns of inheritance. They identify syndromes, support complex decisions, perform prenatal diagnosis, assess patients' risk for diseases such as cancer, and offer genetic counseling about prevention, intervention, and options. They work with patients, families, clinicians, students, and the general public to disseminate the current truth, realizing that today's facts may be different tomorrow, thanks to the rapid pace of research.

Genetic medicine has some unique features that set it apart from other branches of the healing arts. Clinical information involves not only the patient but the patient's living and deceased relatives, the patient's reproductive plans and options, and indeed all future generations that may trace their ancestry back to the patient. Abraham Lincoln is widely believed to have had Marfan syndrome—a genetic problem of the connective tissues, characterized by a lanky body type, long arms and legs, and long feet and hands. A national commission was appointed to consider exhuming Lincoln's remains and testing his DNA for this syndrome. The commission decided against doing so—but Lincoln did have descendants with the syndrome and may well have had this disorder himself. So it is with anyone who has a genetic abnormality: He or she may pass those genes to descendants far in the future. But even in the present, this characteristic of medical genetics makes for some difficult situations. One patient's test results may alter the risks for the patient's relatives. If you are tested for a problem and learn that your children are also at risk, when should they be tested? Who should make that decision?

The power of genetic medicine lies in its capacity for prevention of serious conditions. People with various ancestries can learn the risks they face before they decide to have a baby. Parents can be screened prior to conception to identify specific risks. Prenatal and presymptomatic detection can identify disorders and anomalies, sometimes in time to take preventive steps. The record of prevention in many cases is quite positive. New cases of spina bifida and meningomyelocele, birth anomalies of the spine, have been reduced by simply adding folic acid to the U.S. flour supply and by encouraging reproductive-age women to take a multivitamin with folate prior to conception. The neonatal disorder known as phenylketonuria (PKU), in which untreated children are at risk for severe developmental disabilities, has been prevented, thanks to newborn screening. What was once called cretinism, a condition due to deficient thyroid hormone in the newborn period, has also been virtually eliminated through detection and immediate treatment. Of course, the information provided by genetic testing can be a double-edged sword. A newborn may test positive for cystic fibrosis, and the parents may suddenly realize that their five-year-old son, whom they had been treating for asthma, actually has cystic fibrosis as well.

Medical genetics can also have a dramatic impact on the cost of care. A replacement enzyme that keeps patients with Gaucher disease alive, for example, costs more than $100,000 per patient per year. The cost of genetic testing can be high, and many insurers are still working out their policies concerning coverage, particularly for family members of the insured. Testing for the breast cancer gene, for example, currently costs close to $3,000, partly because the gene was patented by the researchers who sequenced the DNA. The same is true for the evolving practice of gene therapy, except that therapy can be many orders of magnitude more expensive than testing alone.

On the other hand, the financial effects of preventing the development of debilitating illnesses are huge. Whole families can be educated and protected against genetic risks, and genetic consultations can alert patients and their clinicians to prevent even the first symptoms of hereditary problems. Moreover, there are benefits in malpractice risk reduction, decreased human suffering, and improved family communication. There are risks involved in every aspect of medical practice, and some of those risks, particularly in childbirth, are genetic. For example, roughly 3 to 4 of every 100 infants have a birth defect of significant medical or surgical concern. If the obstetrician talks to expectant parents about genetic risks, the parents can understand that the outcome may be less than their dreams. If no one talks to them, they may believe that anything less than perfection is the fault of the obstetrician or the hospital. A frank discussion of risk can build trust and reduce unfounded suits in case an adverse event occurs.

Ethics and Trust in Medical Genetics

The practice of genetics in medicine is ethics in action. Lofty ideals of the "perfect child" clash with the realities of making the best out of terribly difficult situations. A woman with a congenital heart defect faces personal risk in pregnancy, as well as recurrence risk of such birth anomalies in her unborn child. A 36-year-old man, who suffered many surgeries that imperfectly repaired his cleft upper lip and palate, rages against his similarly affected mother for having dared to reproduce. How can he trust prenatal diagnosis to prevent recurrence in the third generation? Genetic medicine raises all the usual medical ethics questions, but several are particularly pressing.

Basic Issues

Like all medical professionals, genetics specialists seek to follow the rule of primum non nocere—first, do no harm. But the harm they can do is often manifested through subtleties such as the tests they order, the information they provide, even the way they frame that information. The 3 to 4 percent of liveborns with birth defects seems much less threatening to expecting parents when they hear that there is also a 96 to 97 percent chance that the baby will *not* have those problems and be well. Clinicians must tell the truth about test results. But how much truth does a patient actually want? Imagine a genetic amniocentesis of a 41-year-old woman that shows an extra chromosome 13 on only one of the cultured fetal cells, that is, trisomy 13 in one cell, with all the others normal. The physician may think the result is no problem, maybe even a lab fluke, and want to ignore it. But if the parents request all of the results, they will worry about that child well into adulthood, wondering when they can be certain that their child is healthy. For the physician, the right course of action is not always clear.

Genetic information that contains bad news can be particularly difficult for a patient to process, partly because it seems so unfair.[1] A person has a disease over which they have little control, and that disease may affect their children and their children's children. Justice, in this context, is a meaningless notion, and patients feel its lack acutely. This puts a premium on the physician's ability to treat patients with honor and respect, to treat patients as the doctors would like to be treated in the same situation. It also puts a premium on unbiased education and risk assessment and on a frank yet caring manner. If the physician explains to patients and family members before genetic testing that the results may contain information that they may not know how to handle, there is more trust available if and when difficult choices must be faced.

Confidentiality

Confidentiality in medicine is never perfect, despite the profession's best efforts and despite laws such as HIPAA. Privacy and confidentiality can be compromised by seemingly trivial errors, such as sending medical records to the wrong fax number. Any physician must remove identifiers when medical charts are used for research and shred unneeded documents.

But genetics raises more difficult issues. A person who gets a DNA test signs a consent form that allows the remainder of the sample to be used for research. This is usually in the fine print, and it stretches the imagination to think that most patients have considered the far-reaching implications. Genetic test results carry information that extends beyond the patient. If a patient undergoes a typical physical examination, the doctor may order a routine anemia test, a hemogram. The test may show that the patient carries thalassemia, a kind of anemia that mostly affects people of Mediterranean, African, and Asian descent, with implications for the patient's family. Yet family members may not want, expect, or appreciate learning that they may also be carriers of this anemia.[2] Presenting a situation that requires perhaps more delicate handling, DNA testing may reveal that the apparent father of a new baby cannot be the biological father, even though he and his wife have comfortably settled into building their new family.

Then, too, the uncertainty surrounding health insurance makes genetic testing potentially hazardous. A patient, concerned about whether he had inherited the breast cancer gene from his mother and her mother, who had both died young of the disease, was concerned for his married daughters. Rather than have them tested, thereby putting their insurability, employability, and self-esteem at risk, he had himself tested at his own expense. Fortunately, the test was negative, and all three daughters were reassured that they were not at increased risk. If the daughters had chosen to be tested directly and learned that they carried the gene, they might have been saddled with the dread words "preexisting condition."

Informed Consent

People want to participate in genetic research, such as research into individual susceptibilities and vulnerabilities to different kinds of medication and treatment, in order to reduce adverse reactions. But consent to the trial must be truly informed, without concern that their care will be jeopardized as they weigh both the risks and the benefits of taking part in a trial.

Signed, informed consent may be indicated when physicians order genetic tests or screening as part of clinical care. To give truly informed consent, any patient must understand what test is being ordered and its potential benefits, the likely and the less likely risks involved, and what will be done with the information. Genetic testing requires that the patient understand additional variables. What is the potential impact of test results on insurability and employability? Is there the possibility that the patient will be somehow stigmatized or discriminated against? What will be the impact of the test results on other family members, and who should inform them? What will the results indicate about the possibility of recurrence? In the case of a child, of course, the parents need to understand the possible disclosure of nonpaternity.

Building Trust in the Physician-Patient Dyad

Patients often present their physicians with issues well beyond their immediate complaints. Some arrive with detailed information from the Web that describes everything about their putative diagnosis, some of it interesting, some quite wrong. Others arrive with virtually no information and often without the language or education necessary to understand what the doctor tells them. Patients often are pressed for time and worried about confidentiality. They are also concerned about whether their insurance will pay for treatment. What if the insurance company cancels their policy due to the illness? What if they don't have insurance? Who will pay the bill? Physicians are often completely unable to allay these concerns. The patient shows up in the physician's office not because patient and physician already know or care about one another, but often because the patient has been referred or because the physician is in a particular health plan's network. The patient is often in some sort of crisis and feels that he or she is in the doctor's office not by choice but by necessity.

What can be done in this situation to build trust? In clinical genetics, the physician has a number of tools available. One practical tool is future projection, that is, helping people imagine future outcomes. For instance, a physician might say, "Let's imagine that you are in the delivery room, and the baby is born. Silence falls. No one wants to be the one to tell you that the baby has the major malformation we had seen on prenatal diagnosis." Thinking through their reaction helps people assess their values and determine an appropriate path; it also helps answer questions about whether they want to do prenatal testing at all. If they feel they could manage the pregnancy outcome, why should they put their fetus at risk with diagnostic tests? How does the hope for reassurance compare to the possibility of raised anxiety? Looking into future scenarios allows them to see what help might be available for them; it allows them to imagine actually being in that situation and then to return to the present, where choice is still possible. It helps potential parents appreciate how close or apart they are in their reactions and values, so they can begin to work on their relationship. Even in cases of illness, such as Huntington's disease, where the future course is uncertain, future projection can help patients and families consider possible pathways and prepare for their options.

Other tools for trust in the front lines of clinical medicine are less specific but hardly less important. Take the concept of *care,* which often seems to have been pressed out of the clinical schedule. Francis Weld Peabody, a pioneering physician, knew that the secret of care for the patient is in caring for the patient. Everybody likes to imagine a small-town doctor who knows you and cares for you—and everybody feels that today's medicine does not allow for that kind of personal care. But a physician can establish a caring relationship, which begins the process of building trust. It starts when you shake hands and say, "How can I help you? I would like to help you." The physician then might say, "What are your questions? Because I want to make sure by the end of the time we have together I have answered them." Another time may have to be scheduled if the list of questions is long. And finally, the physician builds trust by saying, "I want you to call me if you need me. Here is my card." Patients need to know that the doctor is available and that they can call, if necessary. Ironically, people who trust that their physician is available to them often do *not* call, being comforted by the offer of access.

At times, the concept of *faith* can be introduced into the medical office. The information physicians present and the choices the patient faces can be so excruciating that the physician alone cannot provide the guidance the patient needs. Under the conditions of uncertainty, when there is no right or easy answer, clinicians can avoid the conflicts of religion and spirituality by simply asking, "Do you have faith in a higher power? This choice is so painful, you might want to access that power now." Asking this question often helps patients to relax and to find hope. The fact that their physician invoked the value of faith helps to build trust in that relationship.

Another word not often used in the context of medicine is *love*. If a physician can find something to love in the patient he or she is dealing with, if patients can find something to love in the physician, the potential is there for a trusting relationship. Granted, this is difficult to do in a time-constrained appointment. But by finding something wonderful in the patient, we can offer so much more than simple brute facts. We can offer faith, love, and trust, and when the outcome is not what any of us would have wished, we know we have succeeded in the process.

Tools for Developing Trust in Patient Care

The following guidelines are for clinicians who find themselves in the position of dealing with the issues raised by medical genetics.

- *Keep it simple.* The physician is prepared by many years of education and experience. Patients often are not. Synopsize your knowledge and begin with eighth-grade language. Stress causes infantilization, reducing patients' ability to listen to you as an adult.
- *Acknowledge distress.* The patient is in a position of lost choice and control. Therefore, begin by saying, "I understand that this is very stressful; please sit down."
- *Make certain that the patient understands the purpose and implications of testing.* There is no point in jeopardizing the health of a fetus for test results that the potential parents will find neither reassuring nor actionable.
- *Approximate the test accuracy.* Frame the risks in both positive and negative terms.
- *Share decision making.* In a difficult, value-driven choice, be certain to tell the patient that there is no *right* answer, just the best choice they can make, with your help, under difficult conditions of uncertainty.
- *Explain the limits of the test.* Tell what information the test does *not* provide. Patients think amniocentesis tests for all possible fetal problems. It is important to determine what the patient is hoping to learn from the results.

Notes

1. The patient's perception of unfairness increases when the genetic information is given excessive power in predicting a dim outcome. For a discussion on this topic, see A. Surbone, "Genetic Medicine: The Balance Between Science and Morality," *Annals of Oncology* 15, suppl. 1 (2004): i60-i64, esp. i63.

2. Physicians should ensure patient confidentiality, even when the genetic information bears particular significance for the patient's family members. See Rosamond Rhodes, "Confidentiality, Genetic Information, and the Physician-Patient Relationship," *The American Journal of Bioethics* 1 (Summer 2001): 26–28.

IV

Building Trust in the Business of Healthcare

15

Gaining Competitive Advantage in the Healthcare Marketplace by Building Trust

DAVID A. SHORE

First say to yourself what you would be; and then do what you have to do.
—Epictetus (c. 55–135 C.E.)

Trust is the preferred coin of the realm in clinical practice. A high level of trust between doctor and patient improves medical outcomes.[1] It is the best predictor of patient loyalty.[2] Trust is no less valuable in the larger marketplace of healthcare organizations. Is there a hospital, medical center, or managed-care company anywhere that does *not* want to be trusted as a provider of high-quality healthcare? Are there any that do not want to stand out from the pack—to enjoy a competitive advantage—because customers and patients trust it more than they trust the others? Just as trust is good medicine, it is also good business; high levels of trust both further an organization's mission and help build its margin. Indeed, it may not be too much to say that the organization that owns trust owns its marketplace.

So how, then, does an organization build trust among its various constituents? To answer this question, it helps to understand how companies in a variety of industries set themselves apart by creating and maintaining a distinctive reputation. It also helps to consider what might be thought of as the building blocks of trust. Gaining trust is neither automatic nor mysterious. Following Epictetus' advice, it simply requires that an organization do what it must do in order to be what it wants to be.

The Basics of Branding

Many companies sell cars, and most try to sell some other attribute with the vehicle. They sell adventure (Jeep), reliability (Toyota), or status and luxury (Lexus, Mercedes-Benz). One company, Volvo, sells safety. Its cars are engineered for safety. They are designed to look safe. Volvo's target market consists of safety-conscious, affluent car buyers, and the company reinforces the message it sends through all its available channels. Its ads carry safety-related slogans ("Volvo—for life"). Its brochures are printed on thick, durable paper—nothing ephemeral here—and emphasize the company's commitment to safety. The Volvo promise is captured in a quote from its founders: "The guiding principle behind everything we do at Volvo is and must remain safety." It is represented by the first sentence that appears on the Why Volvo? page of the company's Web site: "From the world's first three-point seat belt to the world's first safety concept car, Volvo has set the standard for automotive safety since 1927."[3]

Volvo owns what is known as a *power brand*—a brand that people in a target market will seek out, pay more for, travel farther for, and wait longer for. Power brands are the gold standards of their industries; consumers choose them over competitors because they stand for something distinctive. Disney's theme parks, for example, aren't really in the same category as their competitors. While families might go to Six Flags or a regional amusement park for an evening or a weekend, they will organize entire week-long, thousand-mile trips with the single goal of visiting Disneyland or Disney World. Nor are Wal-Mart's stores in the same category as those of their competitors. Shoppers seeking wide variety and rock-bottom prices know that no other discount house is the equal of Wal-Mart in maintaining well-stocked shelves full of low-priced goods. In the consumer's mind, the distinctiveness of a power brand is emotional as well as rational. Coca-Cola may or may not beat its competitors in blind taste tests. (It often does not.) But people all over the world ask for Coke by name because the product conjures up a host of powerful emotional associations. So it is with many products. Nike doesn't just sell a shoe, it sells the heroism of the dedicated athlete. Fannie Mae doesn't just underwrite mortgages, it sells the "American dream" of home ownership.

There are very few power brands among healthcare service organizations.[4] The one that leaps to everybody's mind, Mayo Clinic, stands out because it is virtually unique.[5] People travel from all over the globe, usually at their own expense, to visit Mayo. In this case, too, the appeal is emotional as well as rational. Mayo doesn't have pharmaceuticals or diagnostic equipment different from those of its competitors. It does have topflight physicians, but so do many other hospitals and medical centers. When patients visit Mayo, they talk not as much about the clinical care as they do about the hotel that is attached to the clinic, the music in the waiting rooms, and all the other features that make them feel comfortable with their choice.

Creating a power brand is essentially a five-step process. This chapter focuses on step number two, building a reputation, because that is the context in which an organization can best focus on building trust. All five steps are first reviewed in sequence.

Raison d'Être

Raison d'être is why the brand exists. It is an organization's mission, vision, and values. Many organizations have mission statements, but it seems to me that a more useful notion is that of a mission *promise*. Volvo promises that all its technology is devoted to making a safe car. Mayo Clinic promises that it will provide the best care to every patient every day. A powerful mission and vision get people excited.[6] When John F. Kennedy said in 1963 that the United States would put a man on the moon before the end of the decade, high school students began enrolling in science courses and planning careers as engineers and astronauts. When Martin Luther King, Jr., said, "I have a dream," people wanted to realize that dream with him. A mission statement does not need to be posted on an organization's Web site or printed in its literature; it is largely intended for internal consumption. It is for the people who staff an organization, the people on whose enthusiasm and commitment the organization depends for success. What should be displayed internally and widely shared externally is the positioning *promise*.

Reputation

This is a key element of brand development. It answers the question, What is the space in the marketplace you want to own? What is the brand's identity in the minds of consumers? What is the reputation you want the organization to have? Marketers call it positioning; you want a reputation that is distinctive, that occupies a unique place in people's minds and hearts. Reputation is extraordinarily important. Coke does not win all those taste tests, Microsoft probably does not have the best operating system, and Maytag, the "dependability people," may not make the most dependable appliances. As long as these companies can maintain their reputations, they maintain their positions in the marketplace. In all likelihood, Mayo Clinic is not the best place to be treated for every conceivable disease. But it is certainly the place that patients think of first when they have been diagnosed with an unusual or intractable illnesses.

Relevance

Maintenance of a power brand requires strict attention to focus. Note, for example, that there are many things that Volvo does not do. It does not produce inexpensive cars aimed at the 22-year-old market. It does not emphasize gas mileage, styling, luxury, or performance. If these features are mentioned at all, they come well behind safety. Nor does Volvo do things like sponsor wrestling tournaments or NASCAR races; instead, it makes a large grant to the journal *Spine* for the best research article. Everything is relevant to the brand's positioning. Chief executives of companies that take their brands seriously think of themselves as stewards of the brands, ensuring that everything the company does is relevant. They often have brand management committees composed of senior executives whose job is to vet everything the institution does and says to see if it is consistent with the brand. When the American Medical Association entered into a commercial venture with Sunbeam Home Health, a venture that the AMA was forced to end after a huge public outcry, someone was not doing this job.

Recognition

Of course, the marketplace has to recognize a brand, and so the brand must be promoted. This is the point where all the traditional marketer's tools—publicity, advertising, communication—become important. But to focus on marketing before taking the first three steps is to jump into the cart, forget the horse altogether, and wonder why it won't move; thus, the adage "The quickest way to kill a brand is to advertise it too much." Advertising needs to be in service of a strong raison d'être and reputation, not in lieu of them.

Repetition

Repetition is necessary for retention; if you want people to retain a message, you must say it over and over, across all available channels of distribution. That's why propaganda is so powerful. If something is repeated often enough, people will remember it, if not believe it. What this means is that an organization's positioning cannot keep changing. Volvo has been selling safety for more than 70 years, and today the marketplace does half of Volvo's work for it. ("You want safety? You should look at a Volvo.") Repetition is the key to the establishment of the message in people's minds.

Building a Reputation

Marketers in other industries know that the key to establishing a power brand is a distinctive reputation. Note that word "distinctive." To stand out, an organization needs something that is unique, proprietary, different from the rest. For years Coca-Cola told us that its secret formula for Coke was more carefully guarded than the formula for the hydrogen bomb. When Wal-Mart was getting started as a national discount house, its everyday-low-prices strategy distinguished it from the repeating pattern of sales and specials that was typical of its competitors. Unfortunately, the need for distinction or uniqueness is utterly lost on many healthcare organizations. Hospitals boast that they are accredited, as if their competitors are not. They trumpet the fact that they have board-certified physicians, as if their competitors do not. Managed care plans are virtually indistinguishable from each other. Some 20 percent of members leave managed care plans every year, and when asked why, they are mystified. A typical response is "Why not?" They see no difference among providers.

Again, what is distinctive about an organization does not have to be tangible or even rational; it can be emotional as well. People buy Nike rather than competitive brands because they want to identify with the sweating heroes in the ads (or just with Michael Jordan). In fact, in studies of marketing effectiveness, emotional benefits regularly outperform rational ones. But whatever it may be, the distinctiveness must be something that matters to the marketplace. Organizations often promote things that make their senior executives feel good: quality ratings, industry awards, testimonials. The buying public may not care about any of these or may regard them simply as the price of doing business. The distinctive feature or features around which an organization builds its reputation must have other characteristics as well.

Consistency

Is the positioning consistent with the mission and vision of the organization? Are all the organization's messages internally consistent? A lack of consistency was precisely what led to the furor over the AMA's 1997 venture with Sunbeam, in which the organization would allow its logo to be used on nine home-health products in return for a royalty. The AMA is a professional organization, not a commercial one, and its reputation until then was as a dispassionate advocate for physicians, patients, and medicine. The commercial arrangement, as the organization's staff quickly discovered, was totally inconsistent with the space the AMA occupied in the minds of its stakeholders and the general public.

Credibility

Is the positioning credible? Can the organization legitimately lay a claim to the space it has staked out? Nordstrom cannot suddenly open a discount house, and Wal-Mart cannot suddenly open a luxury store. The Mayo Clinic can credibly promise to provide the best care; a struggling community hospital's promise to do so might ring hollow. The need for credibility extends internally as well.[7] If managers' and employees' response to a positioning statement is that's a bunch of baloney—that's not who we are, then the positioning is in trouble from the very start. Internal credibility is easily measured, and assessments typically find widespread agreement among staff about whether a particular positioning makes sense.

Scalability and Sustainability

Scalability refers to the scope of marketplace positioning: Can it be applied to everything the organization does? Sustainability refers to the positioning's shelf life. An organization wants its reputation to be built on something that will be just as appealing five or 10 years from now as it is today. For example, Intel's unparalleled reputation for cutting-edge technology and manufacturing excellence informs everything the company does and gives it a distinctive advantage that can last over time.

Putting It into Practice

Let us see how a couple of healthcare organizations have followed these rules in creating their own positioning promises. The Baptist Health System, in Birmingham,

Alabama, competes with an academic medical center—the University of Alabama at Birmingham—and with a HealthSouth proprietary hospital. So Baptist had to come up with a positioning statement that would distinguish it from these two competitors. Here is the result: "When seeking good health, you can trust the Baptist family to minister to your body, mind, and spirit with exceptional care and compassion."

This statement promised emotional benefits—ministering, compassion—as well as rational ones (exceptional care), and it carved out a space in the marketplace to which its competitors could not aspire. Akron Children's Hospital faced a couple of significant challenges. Though well respected, it is not in a big city, and it must compete with institutions such as the Cleveland Clinic. It decided to take advantage of the personal touch and respond to what is always a family member's first question when a child is sick: "Doctor, what would you do if it was your child?" In positioning its statement, Akron Children's promises to work tirelessly on behalf of your child: "You can believe in Children's Hospital to care for your family as we would our own."

Does positioning of this sort work? Fortunately, it is testable. A brand diagnostic study sends researchers out into the marketplace to seek out a dozen or more different stakeholder groups: healthcare organizations, patients, former patients, employees, former employees, referring physicians, volunteers, donors, third-party payers, and community leaders. Researchers ask what the brand stands for in people's minds. They assess whether there is a gap between the organization's positioning and people's perception of it. They measure how effectively the organization is communicating its position. For years, the Kaiser-Permanente Health Plan was seen as the Hyundai of medical care: not too good, not too bad, inexpensive. As Kaiser was transformed into one of the leading health plans in the nation, it had to reposition itself—and it had to make certain that its stakeholders bought into that repositioning.

A Trusted Reputation

Trust is a concept that allows many definitions, but it consists of four key components:

- An unwritten agreement between two or more parties
- for one party to perform a set of agreed-upon activities
- and for the other party to perform a set of agreed-upon activities
- without fear of change from either party.

So defined, trust is obviously a central component of most successful human interactions. In psychoanalyst Erik Erikson's theory of stages of human development, learning to trust is the very first challenge that an infant must meet. Trust is a central theme of literature and ethics, from the bible to the Boy Scout's code of honor ("A scout is trustworthy, loyal, helpful . . ."). Trust is the hallmark of a profession and a professional. The critical component of the definition may be the last—without fear of change from either party. Just as a written contract typically carries a penalty for breaking the contract, the unwritten contract that is trust dissolves into distrust when one party decides to change its mind and do something different.

Trust is particularly important in commercial transactions, in which buyer and seller must have confidence that the other party will do what they say they will do. The importance of trust, moreover, has been growing in today's fast-moving, competitive economy. "A company's trustworthiness, embodied in brand and reputation, is increasingly all that customers, employees, and investors have to rely on," wrote Geoffrey Colvin in *Fortune* magazine.[8] "Our market depends critically on trust—trust in the word of our colleagues, and trust in the word of those with whom we do business," said Alan Greenspan. A certain level of "trust [is] essential to well-functioning markets."[9] Needless to say, trust is particularly important in healthcare. Imagine a two-by-two matrix, with "importance of purchase" along one axis and "degree of consumer knowledge" along the other (Figure 15.1). A few purchases—legal services, financial services, but especially healthcare—go into the box characterized by high importance and low knowledge. It is difficult for patients to judge the quality of the healthcare they receive, because they do not have the necessary professional expertise. Yet, it is critically important that they receive the best care available. Hence, trust is significant. Consumers want to do business with brands that they know and trust. When consumers are patients, they want to be seen and cared for by healthcare providers and organizations that they know and trust.

The importance of trust suggests an immense opportunity for healthcare organizations. The problem described in this book—the general decline in trust in

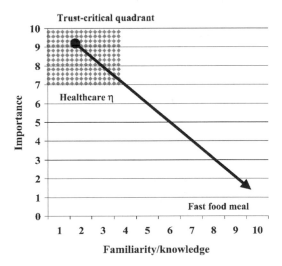

Figure 15.1. Trust brand dependency model
Source: David A. Shore, 2005.

institutions, specifically in healthcare—offers organizations the opportunity to position themselves in the marketplace as the brand people can trust. Doing so can set them apart from the pack along a dimension that is vitally important to the people in their marketplace. It can give them a reputation that colors everything they do and that will last over a long period of time. It allows them to say, in effect, that declining trust in healthcare is not acceptable—and we are taking steps to reverse the decline.

The Power of Trust

It is hard to imagine a more powerful positioning promise. For one thing, trust operates as a kind of mental shorthand. Consumers or patients cannot decide in every instance which doctor they want to see, into which hospital they want to be admitted, which tests they will agree to undergo, or which drugs they will agree to take. The trusted provider is allowed to make these decisions for the patient, time and time again. In healthcare, people always use proxies anyway. If they smell urine in a nursing home, they decide that the quality of the care is low. If the hospital receptionist is surly, they decide that patient care there cannot be very good. Trust is another kind of proxy; it allows people to make judgments that they expect to serve them well, even in the absence of perfect information.

Trust is also iterative and self-reinforcing. If I trust you and you live up to my expectations, I trust you more. Thus, trust builds up over time, which means that the organization that creates a trusted brand can count on sustained trust over lifetimes, even generations. Blue Cross/Blue Shield is one of the few legacy brands in healthcare—brands that have been known and trusted for decades. In Philadelphia, the teachers' union has written into its contract that teachers must be offered a certain type of Blue Cross/Blue Shield product. Just as today's women buy Tide laundry detergent because their mothers and grandmothers did, many of today's patients utilize an insurer or hospital that has been familiar to them since they were children. Although trust builds over time, it can be lost in a heartbeat, if the organization doesn't understand its importance. Enron, Arthur Andersen, Firestone, and even the Roman Catholic Church never quite seemed to realize the fragility of the trust they enjoyed. When they responded to scandal or crisis by trying to cover problems up, trust levels plummeted.

If the organization does understand the importance of maintaining trust, however, it enjoys a kind of halo effect. Johnson & Johnson (J&J), which regularly ranks at the very top of reputation indices in the healthcare products industry, experienced manufacturing problems in a Puerto Rico plant in 2002. Predictably, its stock plunged, from 52 to 38. The next day it was back up to 52. People believed that the company would fix the problem and do the right thing. J&J's actions in the tainted-Tylenol crisis two decades ago are still the stuff of business-school case studies and were voted the best crisis management campaign of the twentieth century. Removing Tylenol from the shelves cost the company millions. But it didn't damage its reputation. Essentially, the company reassured its customers:

We will do whatever it takes to maintain or regain your trust. Soon the sales of Tylenol returned to precrisis levels. High levels of trust allow consumers to forgive an error more readily and to forget it faster. Because every organization makes mistakes, trust provides a valuable reservoir of good will.

As Johnson & Johnson knows, a brand without trust is just a product. In healthcare, a physician without trust is just a technician, and a hospital or clinic without trust is a source of fear. Indeed, 94 percent of consumers say that trust is the single most important variable in choosing a healthcare provider.[10]

The Building Blocks of Trust

So what can an organization do to build a trusted brand, to turn its trademark into a "trustmark?" The first domain of trust is *how people interact.* In a healthcare setting, it is how the physician and every other person who comes into contact with the patient behaves toward the patient. Trust depends on warmth, empathy, and genuineness in this context. If a physician sits down on a bed or comes out into the waiting room and sits down on a couch with a family, he or she is building trust. If the receptionist offers a warm "How may I help you?"—instead of a cold "Your insurance card, please"—he or she is building trust. At Ritz Carlton hotels, a guest might ask a floorman for directions to the ballroom. The chances are good he would say, "I will take you there. It is my pleasure." It is astonishing that so many healthcare institutions, whose very success depends on trust, seem to find it so difficult to learn and repeat such gestures.[11]

The second domain of trust is *integrity.* The brand must deliver truth in advertising. The organization cannot claim to be something that it is not. HealthSouth nearly collapsed because its executives lacked integrity. How could patients in a HealthSouth institution believe that the staff in that particular setting possessed what their corporate bosses obviously did not?

The third domain is *performance.* Warmth, empathy, and genuineness are a necessary first step, but only a first step. Integrity is essential, but it is just one condition for building trust. Performance refers to an organization's ability to do what it says it will do, consistently. In a hospital or clinic, the performance of physicians, nurses, and other clinicians is obviously critical. But so is the performance of everyone else on the staff. Patients who notice overflowing wastebaskets in the restrooms may wonder if the operating rooms are kept clean. Patients who have trouble with their bill are apt to think, "How can I trust the doctors there if the hospital can't even get my bill right?" Good performance yesterday, incidentally, is worth little if an organization's performance today is lacking. The hallmark of good performance is *consistently* good performance.

The fourth domain—the goal of establishing trust, really—is the healthcare organization as *trusted advisor.* Think about the advisors that you have trusted at various times in your life: a teacher or guidance counselor, a priest or rabbi, a parent or relative. You believed that they provided you with advice and counsel that was unvarnished and unbiased, that they had your best interests at heart rather than their own. It is much the same in healthcare. Nurses and pharmacists are consistently among the most trusted professionals in America because they are perceived as operating impartially. Doctors rate relatively high on the trust scale for the same reason—however, the more they are thought to have conflicting interests, as in a managed care situation, the less they are trusted. An organization seeking to be a trusted advisor must be just that: a dispassionate expert. That includes the ability to say no, we are not the best in this field; you should try this provider instead. It involves the ability to offer patients information and recommendations that do not necessarily reflect the organization's interests.

These building blocks of trust cannot be imposed from the top of an organization, though support from the top is indispensable. They must permeate every level and layer, from the neurosurgeon to the parking lot attendant, from the CEO to the housekeeping staff. That is what is meant by scalability. The building blocks must also be durable. An organization cannot use trust as a marketing campaign focus one year and then use a different focus next year. A commitment to trust is like Volvo's commitment to safety. It needs to be repeated year after year, built on and improved upon year after year, until the name of the organization and "trust" become nearly synonymous in people's minds.

Building a power brand, as any owner of one can testify, is a long-term investment. The component of that process that we have focused on in this article, building a reputation, is a long-term process. Trust is not something that consumers give easily, particularly in this day and age. But once they do give it—and once an organization learns how to earn it in everything that it does, consistently—it never goes away.

Notes

1. See for example Felicia Trachtenberg et al., "How Patients' Trust Relates to Their Involvement in Medical Care," *Journal of Family Practice* 54 (2005): 344–352; and Dana G. Safran et al., "Linking Primary Care Performance to Outcomes of Care," *Journal of Family Practice* 47 (1998): 213–220.

2. For examples and discussions on the relationship between trust and patient loyalty, see James W. Peltier, John A. Schibrowsky, and Christopher R. Cochran, "Patient Loyalty that Lasts a Lifetime," *Marketing Health Services* 22, no. 2 (2002): 29–33; and K. C. Warner, "Enhancing Patient Loyalty Through Trust," *Director* 8 (2000). Available: http://www.nadona .org/_state_chapters/michigan/loyaltythroughtrust.htm (accessed April 19, 2006).

3. Available: http://www.volvocars.us/_Tier2/WhyVolvo/ (accessed April 20, 2006).

4. For a discussion on the potential of "power brands" in healthcare, see Michael Petromilli and Dorothy Michalczyk, "Your Most Valuable Asset: Increasing the Value of Your Hospital through Its Brand," *Marketing Health Services* 19, no. 2 (1999): 4–9.

5. For a detailed description of the Mayo Clinic's efforts to build its brand, see Leonard L. Berry and Neeli Bendapudi, "Clueing in Customers," *Harvard Business Review* 81, no. 2 (2003): 100–106, 126.

6. For discussion of branding nonprofit organizations, see Patricia Tan, "Branding down to the Core: Branding for Nonprofits," *Hospital Quarterly* 7, no. 1 (2003): 87–89. Available: http://www.brandchannel.com/features_effect.asp?pf_id=140 (accessed June 10, 2005).

7. For a discussion of the importance of internal brand credibility and how to achieve it, see Colin Mitchell, "Selling the Brand Inside," *Harvard Business Review* 80 (2002): 99–101, 103–105, 126.

8. Geoffrey Colvin, "Tapping the Trust Fund," *Fortune,* April 29, 2002, p. 44.

9. Alan Greenspan, "Federal Reserve Board's Semiannual Monetary Policy Report to the Congress before the Committee on Banking, Housing, and Urban Affairs." U.S. Senate, July 16, 2002. Available: http://www.federalreserve.gov/boarddocs/hh/2002/july/testimony.htm (accessed April 20, 2006).

10. Proprietary study by a major company in the healthcare industry.

11. For a discussion on the lessons that healthcare providers can garner from studying the Ritz-Carlton, see Andrea T. Eliscu, "Ready: How to Keep Your Customers Coming Back," *Medical Group Practice Journal* 47, no. 4 (2000): 46–50, 52, 54; reprinted in Andrea T. Eliscu, *Ready, Set, Market: A Comprehensive Guide to Marketing Your Physician Practice* (Engelwood, Colo.: Medical Group Management Association, 1999).

16

The Changing Relationship between Health Plans and Their Members

CHARLES M. CUTLER

Some years ago, I was involved in a research project studying childhood immunization rates. We asked pediatricians how many of their patients were receiving all of their recommended immunizations by age two. The typical response was "about 90 percent." In fact, as we learned, the rates were often 60 percent or lower.

I think of that study when I am asked to explain what managed care is all about. The physicians didn't know for certain how they were doing but believed that they were doing well, so there was no particular motivation to do better. Today, managed care organizations (MCOs) use a variety of tools to help improve care—for example, by alerting pediatricians to opportunities to increase immunization rates. The result: immunization rates among children covered by MCOs have risen dramatically.[1] By continually assessing how we are doing, we can work to improve care across the board, thereby, in this example, helping to protect the health and well being of millions of children.

Two years ago, the Institute of Medicine outlined six objectives for healthcare: it should be safe, effective, patient-centered, timely, efficient, and equitable.[2] These are essentially the goals of managed care. But two words should be added to this list, "accountable" and "affordable." We cannot know how well we are doing at meeting the objectives, unless we continually measure performance. And the best healthcare in the world will be of limited value if it is priced beyond the reach of most Americans. By striving to make the nation's healthcare system more accountable, MCOs are also working to keep the cost of healthcare broadly affordable for employers and consumers.

Yet managed care's mission has always been controversial, albeit for reasons that have changed over time. The earliest health plans did pioneering work in covering and encouraging preventive care—the then new idea of systematically catching and treating little problems before they become big ones—as well as ongoing care for those with chronic conditions. For this and other things, especially the way they contracted or employed physicians, MCOs were attacked as socialized medicine. Gradually, however, they came to be seen, at least in some quarters, as offering logical ways to organize care and contain costs. Then, in the late 1980s and early 1990s, with the nation's healthcare costs rising at double-digit rates year after year, desperate employers embraced managed care and began to strongly encourage their workers to join health plans. Was all well and good thereafter? Not quite.

Employers expected health plans to save them money, no matter what might be happening in the healthcare sphere, and health plans tried to do so, within reason. At the same time, millions of Americans were making a very rapid transition from one system of coverage to another and in many cases did not understand what health plans were all about. What they heard, incessantly, was that health plans were about cutting costs, period. Soon, it was the accepted belief that health plans' interest was saving money—not prevention, not access, not coordinated care, not evidence-based medicine, not chronic care, not public reporting of performance.

Managed care's critics were quick to exploit opportunities to reinforce consumers' concerns. Arranging coverage and care for millions of new members, while simultaneously striving to contain costs was a major challenge, and some MCO initiatives, no matter how badly needed, meant trouble. For example, health plans' efforts to reduce patients' hospital stays and heavy reliance on emergency rooms, although clinically appropriate, were attacked as ruthless attempts to control costs by denying needed care. To the extent that such changes were put into place without sufficient consumer education, it was inevitable that they would produce a backlash. The media contributed to that, sometimes unwittingly, by using a negative form of shorthand, routinely adding the phrase "whose purpose is to save money," when referring to health maintenance organizations. When you see and hear a phrase often enough, you tend to believe it. People did. Political commentators and Hollywood producers noticed and piled on.[3] It is no wonder that trust eroded.

There is, of course, another side to the story. MCOs have assumed responsibility for managing much of America's healthcare system. To that system, they have brought a new emphasis on transparency and accountability. To ensure that patients get the right care at the right time, information technologies are used to alert patients and physicians to care needs and to measure the quality of care provided. In doing so, MCOs are meeting a clear need. But the need is clear, perhaps, only to those closely familiar with the flaws and failures of the present system. There's the rub. Understandably, few consumers have or want to have that level of expertise. But some familiarity with the evolution of managed care is necessary, so that we can understand how questions of trust have arisen and how they are being addressed.

Historical Roots

Until the 1930s, nearly all Americans paid for their medical care directly. When the first health insurance plans came along, they generally operated on the indemnity model. Patients paid their medical bills and then requested reimbursement from the insurance company. The indemnity model worked reasonably well when healthcare costs were generally low and patients had the funds to pay for services up front. But its major flaws became starkly apparent during the Depression, when even the relatively few patients with insurance were likely to postpone medical care rather than pay for it out of funds needed for basic necessities, such as food and shelter.

Visionary California industrialist Henry Kaiser and visionary California physician Sidney Garfield joined forces in 1938 to create one of the first viable alternatives to the indemnity model. Kaiser, hiring thousands of workers to build the Grand Coulee Dam, asked Garfield to set up a prepaid healthcare plan that would cover preventive care as well as acute care and that would also cover the workers' dependents. The idea was to help people stay healthy and productive, rather than waiting until they became seriously ill and then treating them. The result was a prototype managed care plan that evolved into Kaiser Permanente. Within a few years Henry Kaiser's steel mills and shipyards were powering much of the U.S. war effort on the West Coast during World War II, and Kaiser Permanente (named for one of the mill sites) was growing commensurately, as were other similar prepaid plans.

The indemnity and prepaid group plan models developed essentially side by side, although until the 1970s indemnity plans were much more common and covered far more people than prepaid plans such as Kaiser. Indemnity plans today continue to operate in much the same way. Coverage is determined after a service is provided, and covered services are reimbursed to the patient. The plans typically allow for a substantial deductible or coinsurance, so the patient must pay for a significant portion of his or her healthcare out of pocket. Indemnity plans, which until recently did not cover preventive services, still do not encourage or emphasize that approach to the same degree as prepaid plans. In the original prepaid model, by contrast, the employer paid the plan, and the plan paid physicians on staff to provide proactive healthcare.

These plans proliferated in the 1970s, spurred on by the enactment in 1973 of the federal Health Maintenance Organization (HMO) Act, which required employers with more than a specified numbers of employees to offer at least one staff or group model and one individual practice association (IPA) model HMO (as prepaid group plans came to be called) in addition to traditional indemnity coverage. With concerns about healthcare costs and quality on the rise, HMOs were seen as an alternative that could generate savings by improving the organization and delivery of care. They could focus on and pay for preventive care and help their members stay healthy and save money downstream. They could improve care and outcomes by mounting the kind of thoughtful review of processes and procedures that occurred in many group practices, but doing so over a much larger number of physicians.

Almost from the beginning, however, the rise of managed care organizations was accompanied by confusion about their purposes and functions. Employers, while not uninterested in quality-of-care issues, in many cases were primarily concerned with controlling costs. Physicians, except for those committed to the concept of providing comprehensive care for defined populations, were likely to see managed care organizations mainly as a threat to their independence, their income, or both. Indemnity plans, paying for services after the fact, were not perceived as interfering in the doctor-patient relationship (although once upon a time doctors had resisted them for that very reason). MCOs, in contrast, were seen as a threat to the status quo.

Consumers, even while gaining access to comprehensive coverage and care, could hardly have been immune to the effects of the organized opposition that the rise of MCOs engendered. In many cases the criticism they heard from their doctors was powerfully reinforced by media coverage, which tended to focus less on MCOs' quality-improvement initiatives than on volatile issues such as limits on hospital stays. What got lost in translation was the fact that MCOs were in fact attempting to put into practice the optimal-care guidelines issued by physicians through their professional societies. What came through was the erroneous idea that HMOs existed only to cut costs. In such a climate, trust was perishable—a process helped along by a contentious healthcare political environment.

Managed care in the 1990s did succeed in curbing healthcare costs. Princeton University economist Uwe Reinhardt estimated that the nation's total healthcare bill in 2000, at $1.3 trillion, was some $300 billion lower than it would have been without managed care.[4] In addition to trimming overall costs by some 23 percent, managed care introduced important quality measures and preventive procedures, such as the outreach programs for children with asthma that improved their health and curtailed costly emergency room visits. Managed care brought a new emphasis on performance measurement and accountability to healthcare. Although most consumers consistently reported satisfaction with their health plan, they kept hearing disturbing stories about health plans focusing more on the bottom line than on coverage and care. The bottom line was of no concern to many consumers, because employers were paying most of the bill. The steps being taken to control costs by improving the delivery of care—such as utilization review, technology assessment, dissemination of practice guidelines, and the like—were easily misconstrued as interference and were thus likely to be misunderstood by those consumers who were paying attention.[5] Unfortunately, the one message that got through (reinforced by sheer repetition) was that HMOs were meddling with their healthcare for no good reason.

Great Expectations

In several areas there is a continuing disconnect between what consumers value and how managed care is perceived as functioning.

The Care Your Doctor Recommends

Ask people what are the most important characteristics in a health plan, and the top-ranked feature (after being able to choose your own doctor) is usually the ability to get the care your doctor recommends.[6] In the old days, people kept their medical bills in a shoebox, then submitted them to the insurance company, hoping that some would be reimbursed. Today, the expectation is that everything—whatever the doctor recommends—will be covered. Although the vast majority of claims submitted to MCOs are paid without a problem, there are inevitably times when claims are denied—for example, when a physician recommends a procedure that the plan doesn't cover, isn't adequately supported by a diagnosis, or whose effectiveness hasn't been proven. But when such problems arise, they are often perceived as evidence that health plans won't pay for legitimate expenses and that physicians' hands are tied. Unfortunately, some physicians have used such situations as opportunities to scapegoat health plans for decisions that they themselves preferred to avoid. It is easier to blame a health plan for denying coverage than to tell an insistent patient that a desired diagnostic test or treatment isn't warranted or may not be safe and effective. (This is a problem, incidentally, that is exacerbated by the current fear of malpractice litigation, which drives physicians to order tests and treatments whether appropriate or not.)

Choice

In healthcare, as elsewhere, choice is popular, and the freedom to choose one's healthcare provider is a high priority for most consumers. For health plans, on the other hand, there is a need to ensure that care will be delivered effectively and at reasonable cost, which has meant designing and managing networks of participating physicians. Patients then discovered, in certain cases, that the physicians they preferred were not part of the plan's network. This was a major change and one that engendered much distrust; so much, in fact, that plans have responded to consumer preferences and now offer a range of products promoting choice.[7]

Consumers have also had to confront another aspect of choice. When HMOs were new, employers typically offered at least a couple of HMO alternatives in addition to one or more traditional indemnity plans. Employees could choose among them. As costs continued to rise, however, many employers cut back on the number of health plans that they were willing to offer, creating concerns among employees about whether they were selecting—or being preselected for—the best available health plan. According to one survey, 81 percent of employers and unions expressed confidence that they had chosen the best available health plan to offer their employees or members, but only 62 percent of consumers expressed such confidence.[8] Although surveys showed member satisfaction levels remaining high, this feeling that someone else has made a decision for you is an obvious threat to trust, especially among consumers who, quite understandably, may not take into account the pressure on employers to make difficult decisions to continue providing health benefits at all.

Costs and Quality

In 1998 and 1999, the Employee Benefits Research Institute asked survey respondents whether they believed that healthcare costs had gotten worse in the previous five years. Some 80 percent said "Yes." In fact, during the five-year period ending in 1997, premiums barely increased, the employee share of the premium was essentially stable, and out-of-pocket spending remained low. By most measures, the situation of insured employees had improved, because preventive care was now covered and deductibles and co-insurance were low. And yet people believed that the situation had grown worse. In other words, throughout the 1990s, they were largely unaware of MCOs' effectiveness in helping to extend and sustain coverage by keeping costs within bounds.

As for quality, most patients either do not understand or are unaware of the quality measures that health plans track. If asked what role their health plan plays in assuring quality, most people would probably answer, "None." They believe that quality is exclusively their doctor's job. So one of the major benefits promised and delivered by managed care—tracking the quality and appropriateness of treatment protocols and assessing the effectiveness of physicians and other providers—is largely invisible to the consumer.

Indeed, despite the evolution and increased prevalence of managed care over the past 30 years, unfamiliarity with how it works may be the most stubborn obstacle to trust and the main reason why criticisms of managed care are still so readily believed. Surveys show that most people simply do not know much about managed care. Asked about their familiarity with managed care, only 17 percent of survey respondents in 2002 said they were "extremely" or "very" familiar with it. The largest category by far—as in the previous five years' surveys—was the 59 percent who confessed that they were "not too" or "not at all" familiar with managed care.[9] In another survey, people were asked if they themselves were in managed care plans, and then were asked about the various characteristics of the plans to which they belonged. Most respondents turned out not to know whether they were in a managed care plan or not. Some people with indemnity insurance thought they were in managed care; some people in managed care believed they had indemnity insurance. Confusion reigned.

Strengthening Trust among Members and Patients

"A Changing World Is Forcing Changes on Managed Care." So declared a headline in the *New York Times* in 2001, and it was on point.[10] Managed care organizations have indeed been changing rapidly in recent years. They have been confronting the trust busters—concerns about choice, perceived interference with physician decisions, confusion about access to specialists and emergency care, and so on—in an ongoing effort to address consumers' needs and expectations.

For example, take the issue of choice. From the mid-1990s through 2001, the greatest growth in health plans was preferred provider organizations (PPOs), which allow patients much more choice than older closed-panel models. Experts in the field expect this trend to continue. Or take the belief that health plans were trying to deny access to emergency rooms. This belief has always been based on a misunderstanding. What health plans were really trying to do was to improve care (and, yes, control costs) by steering members to appropriate care venues in nonemergency situations. Today, just about all health plans have adopted a "prudent layperson" standard that says, in essence, that if you are experiencing certain symptoms that would lead you to go to an emergency room, then the visit will be covered.

Similarly, most plans offer open access options as an alternative to requiring patients to go through their primary care physicians in order to see a specialist. More than 80 percent of open access plans allow members to visit any specialist without first obtaining a referral from their primary care physician; the rest require referrals for certain types of specialists, such as neurosurgeons. Even among plans not offering open access, nearly all allow self-referral to certain specialists, such as obstetrician-gynecologists, and most allow self-referral to mental health services. Moreover, a substantial majority of health plans now allow patients to continue seeing the same specialist, even if the specialist leaves the plan's network, at least for a period of time.

Health plans have also worked to address controversies about their formularies—the medications they agree to cover. For instance, a patient might get a prescription from her doctor and go to the pharmacy, only to find that a medicine she believed would cost $10 actually costs $100, because it wasn't included in the formulary. Health plans, I suspect, were counting on physicians and pharmacists to suggest alternatives that *were* included in the formulary, but that didn't always happen. Today, many health plans have moved to more sophisticated formulary designs. For example, some formularies now cover virtually all medications but assign them to tiers requiring varying levels of patient copayments. In tier one, with no copayment or a very low copayment, are preferred drugs, generics, and others that offer good value at relatively low cost. Other drugs are covered in tiers requiring larger co-payments. There are exceptions, of course, in situations where a patient is allergic or is unresponsive to a preferred drug, or for other medical reasons.

Health plans have often been accused of driving down the amount of time that physicians spend with patients. A 1998 study in the *New England Journal of Medicine,* however, found that physicians' time spent with patients actually increased until the mid-1990s and has dropped only slightly since then.[11] Moreover, the study found virtually no difference between the duration of visits covered by managed care and those covered by indemnity insurance: 17.9 minutes on average for the former, 18.5 minutes for the latter. Ironically, MCOs are accused of cutting into patient visits, since under the traditional indemnity model the doctor has a direct financial incentive to squeeze as many patient visits into a day as possible.

At various times in the past, the Harris Poll has asked respondents for suggestions about how to improve the quality and service provided by managed care.[12] Some of the suggestions, such as providing access to medical records, are more properly the province of an individual doctor or group practice than a health plan (unless it is a staff model). But others are measures that health plans are already working to improve. For example, respondents suggested sending reminders for checkups, tests, refills, and shots. Most health plans have been doing this for years. Respondents suggested providing guidance for patients. Health plans are already doing that, notably on their Web sites, with the amount of information (as well as help in using it effectively) steadily increasing. (Many sites also link to online information about services run by leading medical schools, such as Johns Hopkins and Harvard.) Respondents have also suggested working with doctors to improve electronic communications between doctor and patient. Progress in this area has come more slowly than we might wish, however, in part because many physicians are uncomfortable communicating with their patients electronically, even when they are paid for the time involved, and in part because of concerns about protecting confidentiality.

Most important, health plans have done much to improve the quality of care, as indicated by a series of measures. When plans first began looking at the use of beta blockers in cardiac patients, for instance, utilization rates were around 50 percent, and studies show that is where they still are for patients who are not covered by managed care. For MCO patients, however, the number has climbed steadily; the average is now over 90 percent, and several plans have hit 100 percent.[13] Other numbers are similar: the use of Pap smears, 80 percent, cholesterol screening, 77 percent. Even when the figures look low (e.g., controlling blood pressure, 55 percent; controlling cholesterol, 59 percent), they are substantially higher than in the recent past, and higher than for non-MCO patients. Health plans have been equally effective in managing chronic illness. In diabetes care, for instance, 52 percent of MCO patients are now getting diabetic retinal exams, and 80 percent are getting hemoglobin A1C testing. Though there is still much room for improvement, these and other key indicators have all been moving significantly in the right direction.

Information of this kind needs to be broadly disseminated to health plan members. Members need to know that their health plans actively work constructively with physicians in promoting high-quality care, and the numbers prove it. Of course, there is much more to be done. Customer service can always be improved—less time on hold, quicker responses to questions, and so on. Health plans need to continually engage the media in discussing tough issues such as the tradeoff between affordability and coverage. They need to continue to foster a national debate about the underuse and overuse of appropriate care. Stepped-up efforts such as these will go far toward strengthening trust among plan members and patients.

Rebuilding Trust among Providers

To succeed, a health plan must trust the physicians in its network—and the physicians must trust the plan. Moreover, the attitude of physicians toward a plan is a key determinant of how members feel about the plan. In the past, the relationship between MCOs and physicians has often been rocky. At the extremes, plan administrators have viewed providers as inefficient and either unable to understand the rules or unwilling to live with them. For their part, providers have accused MCOs of being inefficient, intrusive, slow to pay claims, and likely to deny tests and treatments arbitrarily.[14]

To move beyond these shopworn stereotypes and improve relations as well as healthcare, MCOs are working on bettering communications with physicians and helping them to improve care, such as by promoting sophisticated electronic information-sharing systems that can reduce medical errors and make physicians' tasks easier. For instance, a number of health plans developed a handheld prescribing tool for physicians, with the plans' various formularies loaded into it, to ease the burden for doctors who contract with plans that have different lists of covered drugs, tiers, and associated cost sharing. Plans are also working to improve coordination of care. Most are operating disease management and case management programs that provide the kind of continuity that non–MCO patients rarely receive. Plans are also making more information available to members about hospitals and physicians and are simplifying paperwork for providers by moving toward more standardized claims procedures and physician credentialing processes. In a number of states, for instance, the Council for Affordable Quality Healthcare has begun a project to collect credentialing information in a centralized database, so that physicians will submit such information for all their health plans only once.

Health plans are currently paying the vast majority of claims within 30 days and often within 14 days, and efforts are under way to speed the process still further, especially when claims are complete and properly coded. (Many doctors seem to think that plans pay late to take advantage of the float, that is, to earn interest on the funds they hold back; in fact, plans would rather pay claims promptly because the cost of delays exceeds anything they might realize on the float.) All plans now accept electronic claims, but there is a need for a standard, easy-to-use electronic claims system. In addition, many plans are developing systems that will allow physicians to check the status of claims online, and some states now have external review processes to which physicians can appeal if they believe a claim isn't being handled fairly.

There is always room for improvement, and health plans are addressing many member and physician concerns. Patients and physicians alike want standardized, easily accessible benefits descriptions so they all know exactly what each plan covers. Many plans are moving in that direction by posting such information on their Web sites. Patients and physicians alike would welcome a faster, simpler approval process, here, too, plans are making progress, for instance, by dropping preauthorization requirements for referrals.

Another topic that has always seemed to provoke vexed reactions is capitation, the system of paying physicians according to the number of plan members on their panel. Critics have argued that, just as fee-for-service medicine encourages physicians to maximize patient visits and scheduled procedures, capitation encourages them to see people less often and to do less for them. Although properly designed capitation arrangements should have no such effect, it is true that capitation has had a troubled history.

Early on, doctors figured that they could do well with capitation contracts because they could manage their patients better than any health plan could. But many medical groups suffered severe losses under these arrangements. Some lacked the financial backing they needed; some lacked stop-loss insurance; some even went out of business. So the number of capitation contracts has declined in recent years, as has the number of physicians who derive part of their income from these contracts. Plans have also grown more sophisticated about capitation. They learned, for instance, that having a capitation contract with the primary care physician (PCP) and a fee-for-service contract with specialists gets the financial incentives wrong; there is no incentive for the PCP not to refer to the specialist, and there is a strong incentive for the specialist to see as many patients as possible. Some plans have therefore switched this system around, so that PCPs are paid on a fee-for-service basis and specialists have capitation agreements.

Employers and health plans are still exploring capitation arrangements. One new approach rewards physicians based on the infrastructure they create. Thus a doctor with an organized registry of patients who have a particular chronic disease would be rewarded, as would a doctor who keeps medical records in electronic format. The idea, obviously, is to drive infrastructure that supports better patient care management. Other plans are experimenting with ways of rewarding physicians for evidence-based, high-quality practice. Of course, any such incentive raises difficult questions. What are the best measures to use in assessing quality? What about risk adjustment? While objective quality assessment is a relatively straightforward process when doctors perform large numbers of similar procedures, it becomes more problematic when doctors manage relatively small numbers of patients with a large variety of illnesses.

Although many physicians have opposed health plans' attempts to assess and reward quality, there is increasing recognition that unacceptably wide variations in practice styles and clinical outcomes—the results of undertreatment, overtreatment, and inappropriate or inadequate treatment—are driving up costs without improving care. My hope is that, over the course of time, most doctors will welcome feedback from health plans and performance measurement as useful tools that help them maintain and enhance their professional stature. Recent studies demonstrate that practice guidelines and disease management protocols are, in fact, becoming more widely accepted—evidence of a willingness to look upon managed care as an ally rather than an adversary.

The Promise of Managed Care

As the national debate about the future of healthcare evolves, there appears to be a rising level of public awareness that coverage and care must be prudently managed if we are to avoid a future in which healthcare is priced beyond the reach of all but the very affluent. Managed care in one form or another is here to stay. As to the question of trust, there is an interesting discrepancy between the results of polls and surveys that still come up largely negative on managed care in general but positive when people are asked whether they are satisfied with their particular health plan. Familiarity, in this case, seems to breed enthusiasm rather than contempt.

Health plans are clearly having some lasting effects on how medicine is practiced and how patients receive care. MCOs have played a major role in moving the healthcare system toward greater accountability and consistency. And there have been significant changes in how the system is used. There is now much less reliance on hospitals for care, for example, than 20 years ago. Without health plans promoting preventive care and early intervention—and asking hard questions about whether so many hospital days were necessary—it is difficult to believe that hospital utilization trends would have been reversed. Other interventions have been assessed for cost-effectiveness as well, and that kind of thinking and decision making is now built into medical schools and training programs. I see this as a very positive trend. Whether you are a physician making a treatment decision or a consumer choosing among coverage options, it simply makes sense to ask about alternatives: Can I get the same—or better—results at more manageable cost?

It is striking to see this kind of thinking, which has always been a core principle of managed care organizations, gaining widespread acceptance throughout the healthcare system. We see it, for example, in all sorts of disease management initiatives—plans and programs that help people to manage chronic illnesses and avoid hospitalization. Patients clearly benefit from proactive disease management, and it is far more cost-effective than letting things go until a hospital stay becomes unavoidable. Indeed, just about all of managed care's core principles, including preventive care, early intervention, coordination of care, continuity of care, and assessment of outcomes as the basis for continual quality improvement, are now broadly accepted as the best way to protect patients and stretch our healthcare dollars in the years ahead. It is ironic that managed care's principles are driving healthcare reform even as efforts to demonize managed care continue.

In effect, managed care made a promise. The promise was to provide access to high quality healthcare at affordable cost and to do it in a way that would earn consumers' trust. To date, managed care has taken the lead in measuring quality and pressing for improved performance; it has kept costs lower than would otherwise have been possible; and most health plan members say they are satisfied with their coverage and care arrangements. That is not a bad track record, especially considering the contentious sociopolitical climate in which health plans operate. And what about trust? In anything as inherently complex and controversial as our healthcare system, trust is bound to be a fragile flower. But if it has been difficult to cultivate at times, there is a good case to be made that, with careful nurturing, it will grow steadily in the years ahead.

Notes

1. National Committee for Quality Assurance, *The State of Healthcare Quality, 2002*. Available: http://www.ncqa.org/sohc2002/ (accessed May 20, 2003).

2. Institute of Medicine, *Crossing the Quality Chasm: A New Health System for the 21st Century* (Washington, D.C.: National Academies Press, 2001).

3. David Mechanic, "The Rise and Fall of Managed Care," *Journal of Health and Social Behavior* 45, suppl. (2004): 76–86.

4. Uwe Reinhardt, "Managed Care Is Still a Good Idea," *Wall Street Journal,* November 17, 1999.

5. David Mechanic, "The Managed Care Backlash: Perceptions and Rhetoric in Health Care Policy and the Potential for Health Care Reform," *Milbank Quarterly* 79 (2001): 35–54, III–IV.

6. Employee Benefits Research Institute, Consumer Health Education Council, and Matthew Greenwald and Associates, *2002 Health Confidence Survey.* Available: http://www .ebri.org/hcs/2002/index.htm (accessed June 8, 2005).

7. For a discussion on the relationship between choice of physicians and trust in health plans, see Rajesh Balkrishnan et al., "Trust in Insurers and Access to Physicians: Associated Enrollee Behaviors and Changes over Time," *Health Services Research* 39 (2004): 813–823; and Christopher B. Forrest et al., "Managed Care, Primary Care, and the Patient-Practitioner Relationship," *Journal of General Internal Medicine* 17 (2002): 270–277. For a survey of health plans' efforts to loosen restrictions, see Debra A. Draper et al., "The Changing Face of Managed Care," *Health Affairs* 21 (2002): 11–23.

8. Matthew Greenwald and Associates, *2002 Health Confidence Survey.*

9. Employee Benefits Research Institute, Consumer Health Education Council, and Matthew Greenwald and Associates, *1998–2002 Health Confidence Surveys.* [Online] Available: http://www.ebri.org/surveys/hcs/ (accessed April 19, 2006).

10. Milt Freudenheim, "A Changing World Is Forcing Changes on Managed Care," *New York Times,* July 2, 2001.

11. David Mechanic, D. D. McAlpine, and Marc Rosenthal, "Are Patients' Office Visits with Physicians Getting Shorter?" *New England Journal of Medicine* 344 (2001): 198.

12. "Beyond the Patients' Bill of Rights: Managed Care Priorities for Reversing the Public Backlash," *Health Care News* 1 (25 Sept. 2001): 27. Available: http://www .harrisinteractive.com/news/newsletters/healthnews/HI_HealthCareNews2001V011_iss27 .pdf (accessed May 23, 2003).

13. National Committee for Quality Assurance, *The State of Healthcare Quality, 2002.* Available: http://www.ncqa.org/sohc2002/ (accessed May 20, 2003).

14. For a sample of provider complaints of managed-care organizations, see Thomas H. Gallagher and W. Levinson, "A Prescription for Protecting the Doctor-Patient Relationship, Part 1" *American Journal of Managed Care* 10, no. 2 (2004); 61–68; and Bradford Kirkman-Liff, "Restoring Trust to Managed Care, Part 2: A Focus on Physicians," *American Journal of Managed Care* 9 (2003): 249–252.

17

Building Trust in a Healthcare System

MICHAEL J. DOWLING

If trust in healthcare is to be restored, leaders of the healthcare industry must take a much more active role in making it happen. This proposition seems self-evident, and you might assume that senior executives of healthcare institutions are already engaged in trust-building activities. Unfortunately, too many healthcare industry leaders are better known for two other activities: complaining that they do not have enough money and lobbying to get more. While most healthcare executives can make a legitimate case for higher reimbursements, we have to be careful about not overdoing it. In the eyes of the public, the outstretched hand succeeds only in undermining trust in the healthcare industry instead of restoring it.

In this chapter, I take a somewhat different approach. Using the experiences of my organization, the North Shore–Long Island Jewish (LIJ) Health System, I discuss what *can* be done to build trust, right now, without more money. I do not contend that reimbursement rates are always fair or that our organization (like any healthcare organization) wouldn't welcome higher levels of income. But it probably makes more sense to focus on issues we can manage (our operations) rather than those over which we have less control (how much we are paid). Of course, I do not suggest that we have done all the right things to rebuild trust; in many areas, our organization is still a work in progress. But I do think that we are on the right track, and that other healthcare leaders may be able to learn from our experience.

Creating a System

The North Shore–Long Island Jewish (LIJ) Health System consists of 15 hospitals, four long-term care facilities, a research institute, five home health agencies, and dozens of outpatient centers across Long Island, New York, and the New York City boroughs of Queens and Staten Island. Its catchment area is roughly 150 miles long and includes more than five million people. Its facilities house more than 6,000 beds and are staffed by about 38,000 employees—the largest employer on Long Island and the ninth largest in New York City. It has approximately 7,000 physicians (including about 1,000 on staff) and 7,000 nurses. Annual revenues are about $4 billion.[1]

However, North Shore–LIJ is not simply a collection of hospitals; it is an integrated healthcare system. Like many health systems, we combined many administrative functions—human resources, finance, planning, marketing, and public relations—following the 1997 merger of North Shore University Hospital in Manhasset and Long Island Jewish Medical Center. Where we have distinguished ourselves is in the area of clinical integration. By building relationships with physicians at both of these tertiary hospitals, we fostered an atmosphere of trust that allowed us to appoint a single chief to oversee the major clinical departments of both campuses. Instead of competing against each other for market share, both hospitals now have the same agenda: providing better quality of care.

Of course, North Shore–LIJ is still in its infancy as a health system. Yet most other large healthcare systems have fallen far short of what we have been able to accomplish during this relatively brief time. Some have dissolved. Others have stayed together but continue to lack cohesiveness, because their staffs don't understand the true meaning of being part of a system. At North Shore–LIJ, five principles have governed the creation of our health system. First, we begin with the premise that all healthcare, like all politics, is local. Now and then a patient seeking care travels away from home, but most go to a local hospital and see a local doctor. Regardless of the size of a system, the people running it can never lose sight of the local nature of healthcare. That is why one of our major efforts has been to build up our community hospitals, which continue to offer a wide range of services. Unlike many healthcare systems, we do not believe that the utility of local community hospitals depends on how many patients they refer to our tertiary hospitals. The community hospitals' job is to keep as many patients as they can and to treat them effectively, close to home.

Second, we have made healthcare quality and patient safety the cornerstones of our health system from day one. When a hospital joins the North Shore-LIJ Health System, all the quality mechanisms and standards that we use in our hospitals are put in place. Each of our hospitals is required to measure its performance using a number of key quality-of-care indicators. On a monthly basis, the comparative data are shared with hospitals throughout the health system. The result has been a significant improvement in quality across the board, particularly in the community hospitals.

For example, a few years ago, quality management data showed that we needed to improve care in the intensive care units, especially for those patients who required mechanical ventilation. Data showed that many of these patients were removing their own ventilator tubes, a nationally recognized quality indicator called unplanned or self-extubation, which can cause injury or complication.[2] A high rate of unplanned extubation raises concerns about quality of care and safety issues. A multidisciplinary task force of quality managers, physicians, pulmonologists, respiratory therapists, nurses, and staff from across the health system developed specific procedures for appropriately weaning patients from ventilators.

This performance improvement initiative had a significant impact on quality and patient safety. Compared with the national benchmark of 10 percent, our health system's unplanned extubation rate is 4.48 percent. By adopting the health system procedure, a newly acquired community hospital reduced its rate of unplanned extubation from 17 percent in 1998 to 5.93 percent in 2002. For the full year 2005, the hospital's rate was 5.13 percent.[3]

Third, we have never made integration itself a goal. This is particularly important when it comes to clinical departments: combining them just for the sake of combining them—or just for the purpose of saving money—undermines trust. On that basis alone, clinical integration won't get the backing of physicians or other staff. But if the goals are to strengthen quality, improve market share, and build a better and stronger system, they will work in a collaborative way to make integration work.

Fourth, we believe strongly in putting the right people in the right places. In this case, the "right" person is the person who not only has the necessary skills but also believes in "we" rather than "I." These are talented, strong-willed individuals who want to work as a team. Those who do not believe in the organization as a whole and the objectives we are trying to realize will not be employed long at North Shore–LIJ.

Finally, building relationships is critically important. The human factor within an organization is often neglected and underestimated. This is another example in which good healthcare is like good politics. Bringing people together, helping them to trust one another, helping them to see their common problems and common goals is how you build a strong foundation for an integrated healthcare system. Of course, it must be done over and over, with new employees and with long-time staff members. It's a never-ending process.

These principles have helped us to build an integrated healthcare system that is gaining the trust of employees and patients alike. We want our patients to always know that they will be treated with competence, dignity, caring, and respect. We want our organization to be perceived as reliable, genuine, and safe. In short, we want to be an organization that not only does things right, but does the right things. This is the essence of trust.

A Focus on Employees

One key to getting there—the most important one, in our view—is to focus on the people who staff the system. The vast majority of North Shore–LIJ's 33,700 employees are nurses, technicians, administrators, housekeepers, bookkeepers, cooks, parking lot attendants, and all the other people who help run a hospital. How important are these people? When patients are in the hospital, they probably see a physician twice a day, when the doctors do their rounds. The rest of the time, the patients' impression of the hospital comes from their interactions with non-clinical staff. In many cases, patients arrive at the hospital through the emergency department, and the first people they see are emergency department staff, only some of whom are doctors. If you want competence, integrity, and all those other trust-building characteristics, you have to rely on your staff to act in ways that support those values. And they must do so consistently over time.

Employees can also serve as ambassadors to potential customers. If we have more than 33,000 people on the payroll, we have 70,000 or 80,000 family members throughout our communities who have a connection to North Shore–LIJ. If our employees trust us, if they feel good about coming to work every day, if they see their work as something more than just a job, imagine the good will that spreads through the community. That kind of goodwill resonates on a day-to-day basis with patients. Numerous studies have shown a direct correlation between employee satisfaction and customer satisfaction. In healthcare, there's no doubt that happy, motivated employees translate into satisfied patients.

Another reason we focus so heavily on employees is because of the dramatic changes that have occurred in the healthcare industry over the past decade or two. Consumers are more educated. They have many options for care, as evidenced by the increased competition among healthcare providers; you can't turn on a radio or television or open a newspaper without hearing or seeing healthcare-related advertisements. Today's healthcare consumer has far different expectations of hospital care. They are no longer willing to wait for hours in a cramped reception area to see a doctor. And they expect to be treated with courtesy and respect, which was not the culture of healthcare workers years ago, and frankly, it continues to be a problem in many healthcare organizations. Some employees continue to act as if they're doing patients a favor by taking care of them. To build public trust in healthcare, it's critical that we change that mindset. Healthcare employees must adapt to today's consumer-focused, competitive environment.

Center for Learning and Innovation

Earning the trust of employees requires more than just lip service; it requires investment, resources, and time. Embracing the "corporate university" concept that has become relatively common among for-profit organizations, the North Shore–LIJ Health System in 2002 created a Center for Learning and Innovation in conjunction with the Harvard School of Public Health and General Electric. The center, the largest of its kind in the healthcare industry, has four essential purposes:

- Create a culture of continuous learning that permeates the organization.
- Foster personal growth among our employees, and provide them with the knowledge, attitude, and skills necessary to support North Shore–LIJ's strategic and business goals.
- Promote leadership at all levels of the organization.
- Create and promote a culture dedicated to excellence, innovation, teamwork, and continuous change.

The Center for Learning, headed by a chief learning officer who reports directly to me, is more than just a typical training program. It's an underlying force of *change momentum* that is driving the future of our organization by totally overhauling our entire approach to human resources.

Education

The beauty of this center is that it offers education programs to people at all levels of the organization. Employees can receive training in everything from how to write a business memo to a six-week Capstone project in which employees learn firsthand how to identify problems and implement new solutions for streamlining business practices. Other offerings include courses on healthcare financing, strategic planning, negotiation and conflict resolution, behavioral interviewing, and how to encourage and challenge employees. The message we send is that everybody needs to be involved in continuous learning. Fostering a culture of lifelong learning allows us to grow as an organization.

Six Sigma

One of the higher-level course offerings through the North Shore–LIJ Center for Learning and Innovation is on Six Sigma, a comprehensive quality program first developed at Motorola and later perfected at many other companies, including General Electric. People involved in the program undergo extensive training in a set of tools and techniques for rooting out errors and faulty procedures. In healthcare, Six Sigma projects can achieve efficiencies such as shorter waiting times for emergency department patients, increased utilization of operating rooms, and reduced time to prepare a hospital bed for a new patient. The program stimulates a great deal of excitement and provides an avenue for the development of new leadership—people who are ready to take on new responsibilities. It helps create a culture in which everyone in the organization is committed to improving the efficiency and effectiveness of their day-to-day operations.

Middle Management

Historically, one of the biggest obstacles to change in any organization has been middle management. Middle managers are critical to any organization; they can make or break a culture change. North Shore–LIJ has 1,150 middle managers, and I personally meet with 70 of them every month for three hours. We discuss values, behaviors, and attitudes. We discuss the importance of our mission and of caring and respect. The middle managers are the people who carry these messages to the troops. Incidentally, these meetings are among many regular employee meetings and social events we hold; there are a number of other, less formal gatherings. For example, I frequently have lunch or dinner with department staffs who have distinguished themselves and deserve recognition. Sometimes, saying thank you for your efforts goes a long way toward building trust and loyalty.

Orientation for New Employees

Every Monday morning, I meet with new employees from the entire organization. It is part of a two-day orientation that typically involves between 35 and 70 people. Meeting new recruits face to face is critically important in an organization as large as ours, and it means a lot to the employees to know that the president and CEO cares enough to spend an hour of his time with them. It allows me to gauge the quality of the people we're bringing into the organization. If you do not attract the right people and transmit the right messages to new employees, by the end of the year you have a couple of hundred new people who may not care about what they do. We assume that the people we hire either have the right skills or that they can quickly learn them. We want to make sure they also have the right attitude and values.

Nursing Recruitment/Retention

The approximately 10,000 nurses at North Shore–LIJ are among the most important employees in the system. Nurses provide roughly 80 percent of the direct care that patients receive. We place a great deal of importance on our nurses and on the quality of care that they deliver. A chief nurse executive reports directly to me and is one of the key people in senior management. We had the first two hospitals in New York State to be honored with the prestigious Magnet Award, the highest recognition that a hospital can receive for its nursing care. In 2005, our health system's vacancy rate in nursing was 3.9 percent. That rate drops significantly when you exclude home care nursing, which has struggled more than hospitals and nursing homes to attract nursing professionals. The vacancy rate at one of our tertiary hospitals has been as low as 1 percent.[4] This is a remarkable accomplishment, considering the national vacancy rate for nurses is more than 13 percent.[5]

One way we have dealt with the nursing shortage is by offering tuition-free assistance to employees interested in becoming nurses. Hundreds responded and most of them made it through our screening process. We then approached local colleges and helped create a nursing degree program in which classes are held at the hospital before or after working hours. Our goal is to graduate 1,000 of our own staff as nurses over the next six years. No one has to sign a form pledging that he or she will stay with us. We believe that most of the new nurses will feel a sense of loyalty to us, but if a few leave after receiving the fully paid education, we will pat ourselves on the back for having improved their career skills. We also offer tuition assistance for nurses seeking advanced degrees.

Service

Hospitals have traditionally focused on the quality of medical care. Of course, medical care is the reason people come to the hospital in the first place. But once they enter our doors, what they experience is not just the care; it is the quality of service that the hospital offers. We want people to experience service that is at the same high level as their medical care. To help make that happen, we have entered into a partnership with The Ritz-Carlton Hotel Company, which is transferring its legendary customer service into our healthcare environment. We believe that patients in a hospital are entitled to the same kind of attention, respect, and courtesy they would receive at a five-star hotel.

Leadership

While we have formalized dozens of initiatives within our Center for Learning and Innovation to foster an environment of professional growth and lifelong learning, there are countless other ways that healthcare leaders can drive cultural change within their organizations. It goes without saying that getting the full support of their management teams is a vital first step.

My senior executives and I spend an enormous amount of time with members of our management team, as well as with physicians. It isn't just meetings, orientations, and events; we also get together socially on a regular basis. Many other managers do the same. Camaraderie and teamwork are essential. As a leader, your job is to create other leaders. It's important to bond with the people who work for your organization, as well as those who don't, such as community and government leaders, board members, and other stakeholders who can influence the success of your organization.

Developing a broad cadre of leaders and building strong constituencies have both been key factors in North Shore–LIJ's success. Our organizational strength has led to significant operational progress that moves us closer to our goal of creating an environment where people come to the hospital, feel they are treated with care and dignity, and want to return the next time they need hospital care. To achieve organizational objectives, every single employee must believe in them and act accordingly. Of course, it's a continuous project, and the messages must be delivered and reinforced on a daily basis.

A few last words on leadership, because without the right leadership none of this will work. A good leader must be vigilant and ready to protect his or her organization against the enemies of trust, which include the following.

- *Self-centered individuals.* Be wary of those who seem more concerned about enhancing their own career aspirations and salaries than helping the organization achieve its vision. More often than not, the benefits to the organization of a self-centered individual's skills and talents will be more than offset by his or her ego.
- *Dishonesty.* Demand truthfulness from your leadership team and insist that they be truthful with those who report to them. This kind of trickle-down effect can cleanse an organization. Without honesty, there's no way you can build a foundation of trust throughout the organization.
- *Inconsistent messages.* Avoid giving mixed signals. Always assume that people within your organization will remember what you've said, written, or done in the past. Leadership comes from the top, and if you want your employees to follow, you have to lead by example. If you have to change course for some reason, acknowledge the change of direction and explain why it's necessary.

There is very little that can stop a group of people who are determined to build a world-class organization and who understand the importance of rallying all employees in that organization behind this mission.

Summary

Regaining the public's trust in the nation's healthcare system requires a commitment on behalf of both physicians and the hospitals in which they practice to break down barriers to change and embrace new concepts. Healthcare organizations must do their part to gain the trust and support of physicians. Many healthcare organizations have failed to provide physicians with the level of support they need to do their jobs effectively. Persistent problems with operating room scheduling, poor physical plants, and unnecessary delays in getting patient test results are just a few of the operational problems at hospitals that hinder physicians.

Hospitals must increase their capacity to care for patients; deliver patient services in a comprehensive, efficient manner; and do whatever else is needed to gain the trust and loyalty of patients. All this helps reinforce a physician's decision to join the medical staff of a hospital. More than anyone, physicians recognize and appreciate working in an environment where quality is held in the highest regard, where nonclinical staff are empowered to improve the efficiency and effectiveness of day-to-day operations, and where patients are treated with the dignity and respect they deserve. The success of any healthcare organization is linked inextricably with the success of its physicians. As a result, the goal of rebuilding trust in our healthcare system can only be achieve if there is close collaboration between the two. Hospital administrators and physicians must continue to prioritize opportunities to learn and to discuss and resolve issues of mutual concern.

Notes

1. North-Shore–Long Island Jewish Health System Annual Report 2005.

2. C. Sessler et.al., "Techniques for Preventing and Managing Unplanned Extubations." *Journal of Critical Illness,* 9 (1994): 609–619.

3. North Shore–LIJ Health System, "Dashboard of Strategic Performance Quality Measures Monthly Reports, 1998–2005." (Internal documents).

4. North Shore–Long Island Jewish Health System, "Nursing Turnover and Vacancy Report, 2005." (Internal document).

5. FitchRatings, "Nursing Shortage Update," May 13, 2003. Available: http://www.fitchratings.com/corporate/reports/report_frame.cfm?rpt_id=172154§or_flag=&market sector=3&detail= (accessed: April 21, 2006). Also see "In Our Hands: How Hospital Leaders Can Build A Thriving Workforce," American Hospital Association, Commission on Workforce for Hospitals and Health Systems, April 2002: 7. Available: http://www.hospitalconnect.com/aha/key_issues/workforce/commission/InOurHands.html (accessed April 21, 2006).

18

Building Trust in the Clinician's Office and at the Bedside

RICHARD TORAN & HOWARD KING

We are practicing physicians who believe trust is encouraged or destroyed every day, day in and day out, in clinical offices and at hospital bedsides around the country. We also believe that trust is not simply a matter of chance or how well a doctor and a patient happen to get along. Rather, there are specific steps physicians can take to build trust into their practices. Because we work in different specialties—Dr. Toran is a neurologist, Dr. King a pediatrician—we have somewhat different approaches to this common goal and somewhat different points to emphasize. Dr. Toran wrote the section on building trust, and Dr. King wrote the section on the patient's emotional life.

The Basics for Building Trust

When building trust, it helps to remember some basics. The first is our means of communication. Our spoken and written language separates us from the rest of the animal kingdom, but the evolutionary trail has been a long one, which accounts for the importance of and our sensitivity to nonverbal communication, or body language. How we behave in the clinical setting and the unspoken signals that we send are as important as what we say. Conveying a sense of caring and competence is essential and takes time. The second basic that is essential to building trust is understanding and always remembering what it means to be a professional, someone who can be depended upon to put the interests of the recipient of a service ahead of his or her own interests. The third basic is adherence to an understandable, common-denominator paradigm of how we help patients (Figure 18.1).

Patients come to us because they have an illness. Their goal is to feel well. The physician's role in helping them attain wellness requires a treatment (Rx), whether advice or an organ transplant. The efficacy of any treatment is dependent

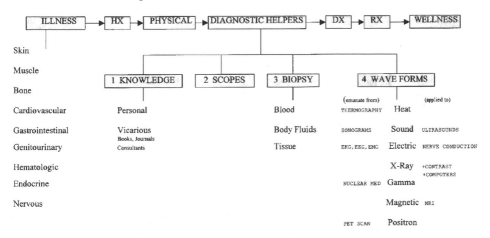

Figure 18.1. Paradigm of patient care

upon the accuracy of the *diagnosis* (Dx), and much of our daily work is concerned with making correct diagnoses. We have only three tools to utilize in making the diagnosis: the patient's history, the physical examination, and diagnostic helpers.

Though this is an age of awe-inspiring technology, the patient history remains our most valuable tool in making a diagnosis. Its usefulness is in direct proportion to the time and effort we spend on it. Much the same can be said for the physical examination. While, the information may be less specific than information received from technological sources, nothing is more sensitive and important. If the history and the physical are not enough for accurate diagnosis, we move on to diagnostic helpers. There are four categories of helpers: knowledge, scopes, biopsy, and wave forms.

- *Knowledge.* The only thing growing faster than medical costs is medical knowledge. At last count there were more than 30 recognized subspecialties for 10 organ systems. Though physicians are constantly building their personal knowledge, they also depend on their colleagues for help in areas that require more expertise. Specialty physicians, by having the luxury of concentrating on illness involving one organ system or category of diseases, should be able to help a patient attain wellness with the fewest number of tests or treatments. Unfortunately, our medical care sometimes seems to involve specialists doing more and more tests. Building trust requires cooperation and communication between primary care physicians and specialists, and it requires specialists to be more oriented to outcomes than to procedures.
- *Scopes.* If history, physical exam, and knowledge don't provide a diagnostic answer, the physical can be extended through the use of scopes. Some scopes are so simple and inexpensive that they are given to medical students by drug companies (stethoscopes). Some—basic but nevertheless chrome-plated—are sold at high cost (ophthalmoscopes). Some are complex and expensive and are used only by specialists (endoscopes). Discretion in their use is essential to building trust.

- *Biopsy.* When necessary for diagnosis, we can subject a tissue sample to a variety of physical and chemical analyses. We most often biopsy the blood, because it is the milieu of all the other organ systems and often reflects their malfunction. Also, it is the easiest to biopsy.
- *Wave forms.* The laws of physics provide us with an array of wave forms that can be used in diagnosis. Some of these emanate from the body (electrocardiography, electromyography, thermography). Most are applied to the body (ultrasound, X-ray, MRI), sometimes with agents that provide contrasts; images from these sources are often generated or enhanced by computers. The pictures are often very high resolution and are invaluable in caring for patients. The drawback is that they are expensive and often overutilized. Building trust in this era of high insurance premiums depends upon patients believing that we are always striving to assure value.

A fourth basic in building trust is a clear understanding and a constant awareness of the environment in which we work. Trust building requires that we appreciate the uncertainties, the hopes, the concerns, the fears, and the demands of our patients. These must always be considered in the light of the state of our healthcare system. At present, it is the high cost of medical care that is eroding trust. If patients understand the reasons for the high cost, we will be better able to work at trust building.

What accounts for the high cost of healthcare? One cost driver is the *technological imperative.* The incredible advances in technology and the improvements in care that they have facilitated benefit both physicians and their patients. Still to be determined is who pays for this powerful technology.

A second cost driver is *pharmaceuticals*—another example of technological prowess that we all appreciate. However, the issues that revolve around pharmaceuticals and drive cost, such as direct advertising to consumers and the desire of many consumers to address all of life's problems with only a pill, cannot be resolved by physicians alone.

A third cost driver is *patient expectations.* Patient expectations are understandably limitless in their hope that we will provide the best treatment, when they become ill. Physicians will continue to do this, assuring value—but if what they do is declared too costly, others must decide who pays.

A fourth cost driver—currently the major one—is *litigation.* A number of factors ensure the persistence of litigation. Patients and families are unwilling to accept some error as a certainty when dealing with illness. A cadre of attorneys is adept at portraying error as malpractice. The attorneys employ the tactic of finding something that might have been done and wasn't. All these have led to an unending quest for certainty. The associated costs are enormous.

A final cost driver is *intern, resident, and fellowship training programs.* All the other drivers—the technological imperative, pharmaceuticals, patient expectations, and litigation—permeate the culture of training programs. As graduates begin practice, these drivers very much increase utilization and costs. We need to set an example in educating physicians of the future concerning the costs and benefits of their decisions and their importance in building trust.

Recommendations for Busy Clinicians

Communicating well, being professional, paying rigorous attention to a paradigm basic to the care of all patients, and a keen awareness of the problems in the environment in which we work are all key to trust building. We wish we could say that these basics are always observed, but it is not so. Since physicians are human beings, they are far from perfect. A startling example of the problem can be found in data presented by the Advisory Board, a national organization that regularly analyzes the state of the American healthcare system. The organization noted the frequency of diagnostic catheterization and angioplasties in a group of 14 cardiologists and 60,000 patients before and after a capitation payment system was implemented (Figure 18.2). Events such as these emphasize the importance of the basics if we are to build trust.

In sum, the following points seem critical for busy clinicians:

- When speaking with patients and families, remember the importance of body language. Be caring. Avoid appearing hurried.
- Develop a thorough and utilitarian low-common-denominator paradigm for approaching illness.
- Keep abreast of developments in the complex environment in which we work.
- Remember what allows the practice of medicine to be called a profession: We put the interest of the recipient of our services ahead of our own.

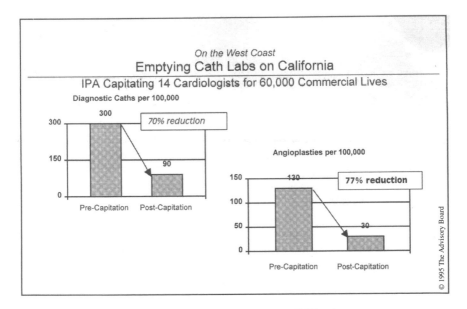

Figure 18.2. On the West Coast: Emptying cath labs on California

Source: J. Z. Avanian, P. J. Hauptman, E. Guadagnoli, *Cardiac Capitation: Vision of the Future for Specialty Care* (Washington, D.C.: The Advisory Board Co., 1995).

The Emotional Life of the Patient

There are many ways whereby physicians could modify the traditional medical model and develop a more sophisticated psychological approach to the average patient and his or her family. If physicians could make use of some of these variations in the clinical interview, the result would be a significant increase in the degree of trust between doctor and patient.

Before we review these variations, let me briefly consider an important barrier to trust: the constraint of time. Most physicians feel obligated to schedule many patients into their day and then feel hurried in the course of seeing these patients. Patients often feel rushed in and rushed out of the examining room. Some managed care requirements don't help matters. Physicians must take the time to explain the benefits of generic drugs, for example, because there is no single formulary created and communicated by health plans. We have to take the time to code our encounters properly and to observe the requirements of HIPAA. With so much time devoted to these issues, is it any wonder that we spend, on the average, only 10 minutes per encounter with patients—and that we typically interrupt our patients 45 seconds into telling their story? The alternatives I outline call upon a different attitude toward the use of time.

First, look upon the entire family as your patient. This is particularly relevant in pediatrics, but it also applies to other specialties. When parents express concerns about their child's emotional health, ask yourself, Who is the real patient? It could be the child in the office, or it could be someone else in the family. The real patient might be one or both of the parents, whose longstanding problems might be surfacing.

It's also appropriate to modify your view of the parent. Traditionally, the parent brings the child to the office, describes the problem to the doctor, and seeks a solution from the doctor. Consider an alternative approach. View the parents as storytellers and as teachers who can help you understand what is truly wrong. Doctors don't need advanced psychological training to employ this approach; all they need is an open mind and some experience with patients. Such an approach also enhances the parents' dignity and makes them more active participants in the process.

Physicians can facilitate the trajectory of parental development. The words "parental development" may have an odd ring to them, but parents have a trajectory of growth and development, just as children do. The key to successful development is helping them improve their sense of competence, for themselves and their children. With the help of the physician, parents can become more effective decision makers, not only for their child but also for their own physical and emotional health.

Physicians can also help parents develop healthier boundaries with their children. No father, for example, wants to project upon his child concerns that properly belong to himself, his difficult father, or his alcoholic brother. The physician should familiarize himself with the parent's history and be aware of how some unresolved conflicts might have originated in the context of his or her own family.

This is not psychotherapy. It is merely approaching the parent psychologically and listening for hidden messages in the parent's story.

The physician should also look upon the child as a potential agent for change in the family situation. The child may be in the office for a routine checkup, but the physician may want to know not only how the child is doing, but also how the family is doing. The child may have behavioral issues, for example, which, in turn, may evolve into an awareness of the parents' seeking help for themselves.

The office visit can become a corrective experience. Process is as important as content: if the physician listens to parents with curiosity, empathy, and support, parents may be able to behave similarly with their children. Many doctors rely heavily on protocols, which is fine. But if the doctor-patient relationship is solid and trusting, even the worst protocol can accomplish more than a great protocol, when the patient is kept at a distance.

Physicians need to inquire about the possibility of family secrets. If we are unaware of past traumatic experiences, we may miss opportunities for constructive intervention. Family secrets might include alcoholism, mental illness, and domestic violence. I see four or five children a month with psychosocial problems, and 90 percent of them come from families in which a parent or a grandparent was an alcoholic. Incidentally, parents don't share this information easily. I explain to them at the beginning of our relationship that these recollections are historically important, and that I won't rush them in and out in 10 minutes. When they say to me, as they sometimes do when they are leaving the office, that there is more that they'd like to discuss with you, suggest that they come back. We've succeeded in persuading local HMOs to reimburse us for an hour's visit that could take place on an evening or weekend day. The telephone isn't ringing, you don't feel rushed, and you can give parents your undivided attention. During that hour or hour and a half, you can explore issues that may go back several generations. There is no way to cover this ground within the traditional medical model. When I worked in an infectious disease hospital, we were expected to diagnose polio or meningitis in 15 minutes. If you carry that culture of speed into dealing with psychosocial issues, you will get nowhere.

It's important to listen for associations. For example, when a parent says, "He reminds me of my cousin Bill." You could reply, "Tell me about Bill—what was he like?" Bill might have attributes that could shed light on a child's behavior. A good question to ask is what are your worst fears? Often a parent might be aware of how a child's actions resembles a relative's behavior and may conclude that the child could become "just like" that relative. If the relative were significantly troubled, that could be very unsettling.

Parents may express an overdetermined description of the child's behavior. The child might actually have colic or an allergy, but they might describe their two-month old as having a terrible temper. To describe an infant in this way is to use words more appropriately describing an adult. It should encourage us to consider that there may be something else on the parents' minds, even if they're not comfortable sharing the story right away.

Parents vary in their ability to talk and think in a psychological way. Some may respond quickly, if you share your thoughts in a tentative and respectful way. Many others aren't ready for it. The best we can do is to let them know that there might be alternative ways of considering the clinical situation. For instance, parents might come in and request an MRI or a blood test because they think the child might have a tumor or colitis, just like some other member of the family once had. You could reply, "I'll be glad to do that test, but while you're waiting for that appointment, why don't you come in and we'll explore this together?"

Many parents provide us with repeated chances to solve these issues. If you give them time, you may discover that they are anxious about their back pain because their parent had a tumor in the spine. The challenge is that we all see patients, or parents, coming in over and over again, often ending up with increased costs without a useful outcome. When patients keep coming back, it is often a good sign that you haven't yet identified the real issues that are troubling them.

Attributes of the physician may become an obstacle to fruitful conversations. Parents may have unconscious attitudes toward physicians, often reflecting how authority figures dealt with them in the past. But physicians, too, may have their own unconscious issues. These need to be acknowledged, because they can affect our ability to listen. It is helpful to find peers or even a therapist with whom we can discuss these issues, which might make it easier to help patients and their families.

When we are stuck, a useful approach is to search for strengths. A parent might come in and ask how they should deal with toilet training or shyness at school. At such times, remind them of how much they have already accomplished in raising their children. I also try to validate their feelings. When a parent acknowledges the pain of past memories, he or she may feel very sad and then apologize for it, as if it is wrong to have those feelings. It helps parents to know that their feelings are legitimate. Even if it is just their anxiety about a child's behavior, the feelings they are experiencing may be perfectly normal. Many times parents have said, astonished, "You mean I'm not crazy?"

On various occasions, it may be advisable to refer a patient to a mental health professional. Making successful referrals is a real accomplishment, given that there is still a stigma attached to mental illness and seeing a psychotherapist. (One child psychiatrist asked me not to put down a diagnosis of adjustment disorder for her child, because she was afraid of what it might mean for his future. She was willing to pay out of pocket to avoid the diagnosis being entered into his permanent record.) Patients need to know that they are not being dumped when they are referred to a therapist. The physician needs to make plain that a referral represents an opportunity for the patient to grow emotionally.

A sophisticated psychosocial approach to treating patients redefines preventive medicine in the context of managed care. The child with a problem may be the health system's first tripwire in identifying a dysfunctional family. It allows health providers to pick up emotional problems earlier, to refer patients when necessary and in a timely way, and even to reduce mental health costs. Early intervention of this sort also helps parents become better decision makers in regard to health and thus become our partners in reducing their healthcare costs. When patients resist taking responsibility—when they keep requesting this or that test, this or that referral—consider saying, "I'll be glad to make the referral, but I also sense a certain anxiety, maybe even distrust, in regard to your healthcare. Can we talk about it so I can help you address this problem?"

Recommendations for Busy Clinicians

In conclusion, let me offer a baker's dozen recommendations:

- Consider the entire family as your patient. The real patient could be another member of the family.
- Provide patients or parents with sufficient time to tell their story, and they will become your best teachers. Doing so also enhances their sense of dignity.
- Help parents improve their ability to make decisions.
- Ask parents about their concerns and worst fears for their child. Ask them about people or events in their family. In the course of their sharing those recollections, you help them focus on their real concerns.
- See the patient as a potential agent for change who could have a salutary effect on other members of the family.
- Invite the patient to a return visit to elaborate their story, if there isn't time in one visit.
- Listen for the overdetermined description. When parents describe a two-month old as having a terrible temper, they are referring to someone else.
- Work with what patients bring to the doctor-patient relationship. Patients, and their parents, vary in their psychological mindedness, that is, their ability to incorporate psychological insights.
- Recognize that patients who keep coming back for further evaluation are presenting you with opportunities to solve their as yet unidentified issues.
- Use the office visit to provide a corrective experience. The physician is still another authority figure with whom the patient must contend. If early authority figures were difficult, an empathic, supportive physician can have a positive influence on the patient.
- Understand your own, unconscious issues. Physicians need support and insight to prevent those issues from intruding into the doctor-patient relationship.
- Remind your patients that they have strengths when they become discouraged, such as how they mastered earlier challenges.
- Refer your patients to a mental health resource tactfully. Inquire about previous negative experiences with counseling, bear in mind the impact of stigma, and help the patient value the referral as an opportunity for personal growth.

One of the best ways to build trust between physician and patient (or parent) is to incorporate a psychosocial approach into the doctor-patient relationship. With time and practice, the modifications described could become a natural part of the physician's armamentarium and increase satisfaction for both the patient and the physician.

19

Conclusion: Trust in Healthcare, Trust in Society

MARC J. ROBERTS

Healthcare costs in America continue to rise, with no end in sight. Aging, new technology, rising incomes—all of these will continue to drive up costs and premiums for the foreseeable future. The one-time savings from managed care have been used up; indeed, those savings are disappearing as a widespread consumer backlash has led many employers to purchase less restrictive insurance plans. Many other employers, meanwhile, are less able to afford premium increases than they were when the economy was booming. Facing less competitive labor markets, they have increasingly moved to pass their rising costs on to employees.

As the middle class begins to experience rising premiums, deductibles, and co-payments, along with decreased coverage, political attention in the United States is beginning to focus on healthcare. Indeed, as companies seek to avoid insurance costs altogether—by outsourcing or by shifting to contract and temporary workers, for example—more and more Americans are finding themselves without affordable insurance. As a result, the whole question of cost-value tradeoffs in the healthcare marketplace is likely to become ever more salient. Price sensitive buyers, corporate or individual, want to be sure that they are getting good care for their money. This is likely to be especially true at the individual level as we move to a world of customer-focused healthcare.

At the same time, consumers are likely to be asked to play a larger role in medical decisions and processes. Some of this change in focus is attributable to the new insurance environment: most doctors and hospitals are covered by most plans, and restrictions on access and referral have decreased, so patients have more choice. Some is a result of consumers having access to more information from the Internet and other sources. Some, too, is due to a growing realization that, in a world of chronic disease, patients are critical members of the care team. They must take medications, alter diets, quit smoking, exercise, and so on. Evolving attitudes among doctors also support this change. They now give patients more information and discretion than ever before. For all these reasons, an age of patient empowerment is upon us.

Together these developments suggest that there will be an increasing role for *trust* as a central feature of every healthcare organization's competitive situation. Organizations that succeed in attracting and retaining patients in this new environment will be those that are most trusted. But what does trust really mean, and how can it be enhanced? Why is trust both so critical and so difficult to create in healthcare, more so than in many other sectors of the economy? How can managers build trust at the organizational level in a way that will lead to competitive advantage? These questions are the subject of this chapter. I first present a broad historical and sociological perspective on trust. What role does trust play in human interactions, and how has that role changed over time? Next, I look at the components of trust—how we rely on the *conscience* and *competence* of others— and how these factors play out in modern medicine. I emphasize the difficulty of clinical decision making on the competence side, and the complexity of physicians' conflicting roles on the conscience side. I conclude with some advice to managers on what they can do about all this.

Let me be clear at the outset, however, that a deeper understanding of these phenomena makes the new challenges seem harder, not easier. Physicians were once quasi-priestly figures with strong personal connections to a much more accepting patient population than we have today. In that context, trust was much easier to establish and maintain, even if it was not always fully justified. In the modern world of cynicism and information technology, the difficulties healthcare managers and providers confront are much more formidable. They cannot be dealt with successfully, however, unless we first recognize their nature and origins.

The Evolving Role of Trust

The capacity for and the need to trust are rooted in our evolutionary experience. Our ancestors on the plains of East Africa were relatively weak, slow creatures who could not come close to matching antelopes for speed, lions for strength, or elephants for bulk. For survival, they had to cooperate. Achieving that cooperation required trust.

Trust even then had two components. Since much work was shared, early humans had to trust the *competence* of their companions. If some drove game toward others in the band, they had to believe that the hunt would conclude successfully. If some picked fruits for the group, the rest had to trust the pickers to tell the edible from the harmful. Our distant ancestors also had to trust that other members of the group would follow social norms including obeying the dictates of *conscience* as constructed by their culture. If I am to bring all that I have gathered to a common meal, I have to trust that others will do likewise. When others stand guard at night, I have to trust that they will be vigilant and not kill me in my sleep because they covet some prized possession—or my spouse.

In a primitive band, everyone learned quickly who could be trusted. Competence and conscience were repeatedly revealed through face-to-face interactions. Norms were likely to be ruthlessly enforced, since untrustworthy behavior seriously affected everyone's life expectancy. No wonder modern humans are so strongly programmed to follow social norms. Those among our ancestors who were not hardwired in this way undoubtedly enjoyed noticeably less reproductive success.

Until the second half of the nineteenth century, most people lived in a world dominated by interactions with known others: local craftsmen, nearby storekeepers, neighbors, and friends. Only with the rise of the telegraph, steamship, railroad, and mass production did it become possible and profitable to operate companies on a regional or national scale. The early rise of brand names reflects that transformation; brands are a way of establishing trust with a mass of anonymous customers.

In recent decades, we have seen a comparable transformation of the retail sector. Metropolitan highway systems have created metropolitan retail markets, often driving the neighborhood drugstore, hardware store, bank, or hospital out of business. The rise of regional and national media, especially television, has created economies of scale in advertising, disadvantaging small sellers still further and leading to an ever greater salience for branding.

Still more recently, new information technology and ever improving transportation have made possible national and international purchasing and distribution. Now everyone in America can go to a mall with a Gap, Pottery Barn, Kmart, Staples, or Target. (Notice that all of these are well-known brands.) As transportation improvements and lowered trade barriers have created more and more worldwide markets, many countries now complain about the cultural imperialism of Levi's, Coca-Cola, McDonald's, American television shows, and the global capitalism these represent.

Trust in Healthcare

Nowhere in the modern world is trust more important than in healthcare. This is because the patient-as-customer often has to rely on the doctor-as-seller to determine what the patient should purchase. The doctor must act as the patient's agent. Yet doctors face other incentives. Fee-for-service reimbursement gives them reason to do more, while a salaried position without performance incentives gives them reason to do less. The conflicts of interest inherent in such an agency relationship can only be overcome by trust.

Trust in this context depends on doctors following professional norms even at the expense of their own self-interest. Yet external pressures can erode the constraints of conscience. In recent years, for instance, many Chinese doctors have been given bonuses by their hospitals, reflecting the profits they generate from prescribing drugs. (Hospitals in China sell drugs directly to patients.) This, in turn, has lead to well-documented patterns of drug overuse. Conversely, nephrologists in the

United Kingdom, who have limited dialysis capacity at their disposal, are much quicker than their U.S. counterparts to decide that older patients are not appropriate candidates for such treatment. In the United States, the rise of managed care has led many to question whether the financial interests of doctors or the limits put on them by insurance companies are likewise influencing how they use their power within their agency relationships.

Just as patients have to trust their doctor's conscience, they also must trust their competence. But competence is difficult for them to judge. For most patients, most of the time, judgments about clinical quality remain elusive. The fact that, in England, a Yorkshire general practitioner could murder more than 200 of his patients while becoming a respected community figure only attests to such problems. (Talk about being unable to recognize poor quality of care!) Instead, patients often rely on *service* quality (e.g., amenities, interpersonal treatment, etc.) as a proxy for clinical quality. Only in seriously underfunded situations (e.g., health centers in poor countries that lack basic medications) are clinical quality problems likely to be directly evident to patients. In rich countries, patients often use quantity of care as a proxy for quality. But someone who says, "Grandma got high-quality care—they did everything for her," cannot usually tell whether everything was done well or badly.

However they are made, patients' judgments about quality are also based on their expectations. These expectations vary both within and across nations. American patients have very high expectations, reflected in the popular quip that medical science has made death optional. Media portrayals of heroic doctors, widespread gee-whiz media coverage of new scientific developments, pervasive pharmaceutical advertising, and years of public advocacy for causes such as National Institutes of Health budgets have all left their mark. In a culture with an optimistic bias and a broad faith in science and technology, these pressures in the direction of higher expectations have found a strong response in popular beliefs. As a result, Americans now want and expect to get prompt and unlimited access to the latest technology with little or no out-of-pocket cost. Only the best will do, even as consumers' actual capacity to evaluate competence remains quite limited.

Medical Science and the Difficulties of Clinical Practice

The difficulties consumers have in judging medical competence are exacerbated by the nature of medical practice. The same difficulties hamper the efforts of managers who want to build trust among their patients by ensuring that they receive competent care. Medicine is still largely a craft informed by science. We know a good deal about anatomy and physiology and about the molecular biology of many diseases. But that does not mean that medical science has a well-supported therapeutic response for every disease or condition. Much of the evolution of clinical practice has been based on intuition or judgment without rigorous evaluation. And that intuition or judgment, however plausible, can turn out to be mistaken.

There are many, many examples. Recently, hormone replacement therapy, long seen as a panacea for everything from menopause to heart disease, has been shown to increase the risk for heart disease rather than decrease it. Similarly, high-dose chemotherapy together with bone marrow transplant, an extremely stressful and risky procedure, has proved not to improve the survival of metastatic breast cancer patients. In the more distant past, one could find examples such as bleeding with leeches, freezing as a treatment for gastric ulcers, and the unforeseen side effects of various diet drugs.

These mistakes are rooted in the nature of medical practice. Human beings have an enormous capacity to survive without clinical care. Since we have had effective medicine for only 70 or 80 years, we never would have populated the planet if this were not so. This means that, except for those with the most acute illnesses, most patients recover, provided the care we give is not too injurious. Hence, even poor practices can seem beneficial to an individual practitioner. Most of the tens of thousands of fever patients who were bled in the seventeenth and eighteenth centuries survived, which only convinced their physicians of the efficacy of this treatment. Also consider the placebo effect. Because the body and mind are connected, a patient's faith in a treatment often makes the patient feel better, even when there is no biological reason for the improvement. Again, a practitioner's experience is likely to be deceptively optimistic.

To truly test whether a treatment is effective requires a large, well-designed study. We need large numbers to detect the modest impact that most treatments actually provide. We need control groups to see what happens in the absence of care. We may need random assignment of patients to treatment options to guard against selection bias. And we need a double-blind design, in which neither patients nor doctors know who has received which intervention, to prevent placebo effects.

Such studies are difficult and expensive to conduct, and in fact they have never been carried out for many widely accepted therapeutic options. This situation means that doctors' clinical judgments about correct care can be seriously flawed, even as the doctors become more deeply committed to them. Real clinical research is well beyond the capacity of an individual practitioner. Most doctors see small numbers of any one kind of patient and treat them without the benefit of control groups or random assignment. Moreover, doctors are likely to remember their successes more than their failures. No wonder so many doctors continue to provide inappropriate care too long.

The psychology of medical training and practice only reinforces practitioners' resistance to changing their clinical decisions. Medicine is still taught in an apprenticeship mode. Young doctors come under the influence of senior practitioners who pass on their particular patterns of treatment. Young doctors-in-training have enormous responsibilities, often involving life and death. The anxiety such responsibility provokes can be managed only if one believes in what one has been taught and in one's own capacity to apply it case by case. As a result, clinicians can become quite defensive and entrenched in their opinions, regardless of the data. Comments like "That is not how I was taught," "My patients are different," and "My clinical judgment tells me otherwise," are common reactions to efforts to persuade doctors to change their approach to care.

The difficulties of clinical practice also play a role. Human beings are remarkably variable. One patient will react well to one drug and not to another, while a second individual exhibits the opposite pattern. So even where well-designed clinical trials are available, the results need to be applied to patients with judgment based on experience. After all, the relevant study might have been done on 50-year-old Finnish men without complications, and your patient is a 65-year-old African-American woman with multiple diagnoses.

The Difficulties of Managing Medical Decisions

The scientific difficulties of ensuring clinical competence intersect with a set of managerial difficulties that make it difficult for organizations to build a quality reputation that they genuinely deserve and hence to earn trust at the institutional level. Patients suffer from hundreds of different diseases and conditions. Medical practice consists of a large number of individually small, highly varied decisions and activities. The individual practitioners who make these decisions and engage in these activities resist efforts to limit their autonomy.

All this makes it very difficult to measure and monitor the quality of clinical care at the level of the individual provider. With the exception of some highly specialized practitioners (e.g., high-volume cardiac surgeons), most providers see too few patients of any one type for them to be judged by the outcomes of their care. Where accepted clinical guidelines exist, conformance to process standards can be monitored as a quality control technique. But the degree of patient variation, the limited availability of such guidelines, and doctors' unwillingness to accept them make such efforts relatively difficult. Moreover, the record review that is required by these process controls can be taxing, except in those (still unusual) cases where there are extensive electronic records.

Contrast this managerial dilemma with the problems of quality control in a large corporate law firm. The law firm has even less reliable science to rely on than does medicine. But it focuses on a much smaller number of cases. Each lawyer doesn't see dozens of new clients each week. A team handles each case, with senior partners providing detailed supervision and review of more junior members' decisions. Lawyers give much more attention to each case (typically adding up hundreds of billable hours). There is much discussion and much peer review.

In medicine, by contrast, the need for judgment and craft, together with the need for belief in one's own choices, has led to a culture that places great emphasis on the autonomy of individual doctors. Physicians and surgeons are reluctant to second-guess each other's decisions. There is a widespread, implicit "mutual nonaggression pact" that serves most practitioners' interests. It implies the promise "I won't question your clinical decisions if you don't question mine." As a result, disciplinary bodies under the auspices of medical societies are reluctant to pursue any but the most flagrant offenses. Indeed for many years, testifying against another physician in a malpractice case was a violation of the AMA's Code of Ethics. Similarly, when nonphysician managers urge error reduction or process-improvement efforts, they are often met with a mixture of hostility and contempt—"You are not a doctor. It's no wonder you don't understand."

Problems of Conscience

Managers who want to build trust in their organizations must deal with issues of conscience as well as competence. Here the fundamental dilemma is that doctors have to fulfill at least *five* conflicting roles, and the demands of conscience vary across these roles. This can lead to serious internal conflicts for even the most conscientious physician. Managers who want to lead a trustworthy organization must find a way to guide their employees through these conflicting demands. The roles and their respective imperatives include the following.

- *Caregiver.* Respond to patients' expectations and desires. Provide emotional support to help them deal with the psychological burden of disease.
- *Clinical expert.* Provide the best possible treatment, that is, care that meets consensus standards of what is appropriate.
- *Organization member.* Respond to the organization's policies and priorities; act to advance the organization's interests.
- *Economic actor.* Respond to one's incentives and interests. Maximize one's economic welfare.
- *Citizen/moral actor.* Make decisions that are socially responsible and morally defensible.

The point of this typology is that the traditional economic analysis of the "agency problem" is too simple. It typically depicts the issue as a tension between *clinical expert* and *economic actor.* In fact the conflicts that arise for doctors in the modern world are much more complex. Patients can desperately want and be willing to pay for therapy that is clinically unnecessary and socially irresponsible (e.g., antibiotics for viral respiratory infections, surgery for cancer that is too advanced for the procedure to do much good). Organizations can ask their members to make individual sacrifices for the collective good or to distort their clinical choices to advance the organization's interest. Any or all of these points of views can lead to decisions that some would find irresponsible, even morally indefensible. How, then, is a physician to act conscientiously? What does it even mean for a manager to try to develop adherence to such patterns of behavior within his or her organization?

Here is a true minicase that illustrates these points. Imagine that you are the doctor running an emergency room (ER) in a downtown academic hospital in a large city, where you have several significant competitors. The decision you must make is when to signal the city's emergency medical team (EMT) service that you are at capacity and that they should divert patients to other institutions. Among the salient facts are the following: Your hospital is in serious financial trouble. Many trauma patients are uninsured. Because of nursing shortages, ER patients at your hospital have to wait up to 24 hours for a bed. Your fiscally healthier competitors close their ERs frequently. Smaller suburban hospitals, which "med flight" complex cases, are more likely to send you uninsured rather than insured patients. Finally, according to your contract with the hospital, your income goes up when you treat more patients, regardless of their insurance status.

So when things get busy, what do you do? To make things more complex, suppose that an insured patient whose doctor is on the hospital's staff telephones when you are on diversion. Do you tell the patient to come in anyway? How do you balance concern for the patients, concern for the hospital, social responsibility, and your own financial interests? To push the question still further, do you have any obligation to press the hospital to expand its ER capacity? Do you have any obligation to go to the Department of Health to get new rules passed to standardize diversion decisions for hospitals and perhaps constrain your competitors? How much time and energy should the chief ER doctor devote to those tasks versus improving the quality of care for the patients who come through the door? Moreover, should your behavior change once the hospital's financial situation improves? What does it mean to act in a trustworthy manner in such situations?

Possible Responses: Trust through Competence

The first set of tasks faced by a manager who wants to build trust is to achieve genuine competence in the organization. That is the way to earn and deserve trust on this dimension. And this means managing the process of clinical care, however difficult.

The key here is to focus on care systems; to engineer these systems so that it is easy to do things well and hard to do them wrong. A study of the relative reliability of air conditioners found that the manufacturer with the best performance had achieved it by intelligent design. The various electrical connections, hoses, and so forth, in their units had been sized and shaped so that it was almost impossible to assemble the machines incorrectly.

In hospitals, we know a lot about the sources of human error (e.g., stress, distraction, sleeplessness, etc.), and we could improve quality significantly by figuring out how to minimize or work around such factors. If nurses make medication errors when they can't read a doctor's handwriting, for instance, we can implement computerized order entry. If overstressed surgeons get confused about which limb to operate on, we can have them "sign the site" in peace and quiet, with an awake patient, the day before surgery. Real process improvement requires managers to take errors seriously and to remember the quality maxim "Every complaint is a jewel." When errors are detected, managers need to look for solutions, not scapegoats. Organizations even need to encourage and reward internal whistle blowers who alert their superiors to developing problems.

An ironic but useful counterpart to doing better is to develop more realistic expectations among customers. Customers judge performance by the gap between what they perceive and what they expect. Improving real performance may well improve perceived performance, and if perception lags behind reality, better communication can help. In addition, lowering expectations may play a useful role. One hospital ER installed an electronic sign that displayed frequently updated estimates of waiting times; it experienced a large decrease in complaints about such waits, even without improving performance. Every experienced restaurant maître d' uses the same approach.

Given the nature and limits of medical science and given the deep commitment to autonomy at the core of U.S. physicians' professional culture, following this program will not be easy. Doctors will resist algorithms and protocols. They will see system change as someone else's job (e.g., nurses, managers, etc.). Although developments in information technology are making the task easier, and although younger doctors are entering practice with slightly different expectations, there is much difficult work to be done here. Still, the very fact that trust in medical care and in doctors seems to be declining in the United States makes such efforts that much more attractive from a competitive point of view. If all patients thought that all doctors were wonderful, there would be much less room for developing product differentiation and distinctive competence in the quality arena. The few national brand names in healthcare, such as Mayo Clinic, are perceived as providing reliably high clinical quality.

Possible Responses: Trust through Conscience

Given the complex conflicts that trouble healthcare providers, the first task for responsible managers is to acknowledge this reality, both internally and externally. A reputation for acting in good conscience can be earned only by fostering transparency and accountability. The first step down such a road is to take an honest account of the situation.

In a way, the simplest advice to give managers concerns crisis management. The undoubted truth that the cover-up is worse than the crime is a wise guide here. Even victims of mistakes often are not focused primarily on imposing punishment on those who erred. Instead, they may care more about hearing an acknowledgment of their troubles, receiving an apology, and being assured that corrective action is being taken so that mistakes like the one that injured them will be prevented from happening in the future. Telling the truth and acting aggressively to improve processes is clearly the right advice for managers in such situations.

But what can managers do to build trust through routine operations? One place to begin is to write mission and vision statements that convey to both employees and patients how the organization intends to deal with the tensions it confronts between mission and margin. The organization can then devise a strategy that responds to the need for such balance. It can develop a set of policies and practices that are consistent with its stated goals and linked to them in an explicit fashion. Internal arrangements, like the incentive and compensation plans for employees (including physicians) can then be crafted to align those incentives with the strategic priorities. Employees can be trained to recognize and respond to the conflicting demands of conscience raised by their multiple roles in a self-aware and honest way.

Through all this, managers also need to find ways to be more accountable. It is worth repeating: transparency and accountability build trust. That is one of the ironies of the reaction of the accounting profession to the recent wave of corporate accounting scandals. Rather than resisting tough disclosure standards, the largest firms would be wiser to welcome them. The more open the disclosure, the more the public will feel able to trust the products of what has become, for many, a highly untrustworthy set of institutions.

Stepping Up to the Future

These challenges present difficult decisions for all in the healthcare system: patients and providers, payers and managers. *Patients* are likely to continue to want unlimited and convenient access to services with no financial or procedural barriers, even as they complain about the increases in their healthcare costs. *Physicians* are likely to resist what they see as a loss of their professional autonomy, even as they resist efforts to get them to take collective responsibility for controlling costs and improving the quality of care. *Payers* will ask patients to make quality judgments that the payers themselves are unable to make and then will complain about the failure of the market to exert effective discipline. *Managers* will despair over the unwillingness of physicians to cooperate in the task of responsible resource use, even as they avoid direct confrontation with physicians that might provoke a more honest discussion.

If we are to lower current unrealistic expectations and improve our current, often highly imperfect, performance simultaneously, something will have to change. Academic physicians must take the lead in defining appropriate care. Teamwork among the various professions in a hospital—doctors, nurses, managers, and so on—will have to increase. A new culture of transparency and accountability will have to develop. Only then will we have a twenty-first-century healthcare system worthy of the trust of a twenty-first-century population. Those in the industry who move first and most aggressively in these directions, I believe, could find the rewards even greater than the admittedly significant difficulties that will attend such trust-building endeavors.

Index

Page numbers in italic indicate figures, those in bold are tables. Endnotes numbers follow the page number, such as 19n35.